Sally Gainsbury

Internet Gambling

Current Research Findings and Implications

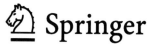 Springer

Sally Gainsbury
Southern Cross University
Lismore, NSW, Australia

ISSN 2192-2888   e-ISSN 2192-2896
ISBN 978-1-4614-3389-7   e-ISBN 978-1-4614-3390-3
DOI 10.1007/978-1-4614-3390-3
Springer New York Dordrecht Heidelberg London

Library of Congress Control Number: 2012932207

Springer is part of Springer Science+Business Media (www.springer.com)

Contents

Chapter 1
Introduction

Abstract Internet gambling is a rapidly evolving mode of gambling and increasingly recognized by researchers, policy makers, industry groups, and community groups as having a substantial impact on society. Beginning as a handful of online casinos in the Caribbean, the industry has undergone a remarkable transformation with a period of rapid expansion followed by consolidation. A highly competitive market now exists based on sophisticated technology and increasingly informed and demanding consumers. There is clear evidence that Internet gambling participation and revenue are increasing, and many policies and regulations currently in place are ineffective. Internet gambling has distinct characteristics that differentiate it from traditional land-based gambling and appeal to new markets. These features pose both challenges and opportunities and it is essential that researchers, industry and government act to respond to Internet gambling and the numerous related social issues. This chapter provides an overview of the online gambling market and introduces key points that are essential to understanding the growth of and impact of this new mode of gambling.

Keywords Internet gambling • Online gaming • Policy • Driving factors • Market • Impacts

Internet gambling is a rapidly evolving mode of gambling and increasingly recognized by researchers, policy makers, industry groups, and community groups as having a substantial impact on society. The term Internet gambling is often used interchangeably with online gambling and refers to all forms of gambling (including wagering) via the Internet, including gambling using computers, mobile phones or wireless devices connected to the Internet. Interactive gambling is a slightly broader term, although again often used interchangeably with Internet gambling, and includes other forms of remote gambling generally conducted via digital means such as digital television. This definition exists with the generally accepted definition of gambling activities as involving wagering a stake with monetary value in games in which the

S. Gainsbury, *Internet Gambling: Current Research Findings and Implications*,
SpringerBriefs in Behavioral Medicine 1, DOI 10.1007/978-1-4614-3390-3_1,
© Springer Science+Business Media, LLC 2012

outcome is determined by chance. Internet, and other interactive technological platforms, are used to (a) offer gambling services to consumers, (b) allow consumers to bet or gamble against each other, for example betting exchanges or online poker, of (c) as a distribution technique, for example to purchase lottery tickets online (European Commission 2011a).

Following the growth of personal and high speed computers the commercialization and development of Internet Services Providers in the 1980s saw increased growth amongst the general population. Gambling sites began to appear in the 1990s. The earliest confirmed date for an authentic Internet gambling site is September, 1993 when the Swiss Lottery (Loterie Romande) began selling lottery tickets to individuals with a special terminal and software (Pavalko 2004). In 1994, the Antiguan government passed legislation permitting online casinos to be established. Intercasino was the first online casino to accept real money wagers, launched in Antigua in 1996 (it is now registered in Malta) and their revenue reports attracted significant interest.

Since the early beginnings of Internet gambling, the number of online gambling sites has increased at an astounding rate each year. In 1994 there were reportedly 30 gambling websites (Swartz 2005) but 4 years later, there were approximately 90 online casinos, 39 lotteries, 8 online sites offering bingo, and 53 sports books (Basham and White 2002). By 1999, the number dramatically increased to 250 online casinos, 64 lotteries, 20 bingo and 139 sports books (Auriemma and Lahey 1999; Basham and White 2002). In the 1990s, Internet gambling operators largely focussed on the North American market with private sites licensed in the Caribbean; after 2001 European and offshore licenses saw Internet gambling expand globally, with a mix of public and private companies eventually looking towards markets in the US and Asia (Holliday 2011).

Since the initial explosive market expansion, it appears that the increase in number of sites has somewhat tapered off as larger companies purchase smaller sites and the market consolidates. It was estimated that there were approximately 2,300 online gambling sites in 2006 (Ranade et al. 2006), a number similar to the 2,485 sites estimated to be available in July 2011 (Casino City 2011). The majority of these sites are privately owned and there are 666 different companies regulated in 75 jurisdictions (Casino City 2011). The current Internet gambling market includes 770 casino sites, 590 poker sites, 433 sports and racebooks, 401 bingo sites, 106 lottery sites and a variety of skill games and betting exchanges.

Participation in Internet gambling is still relatively low compared to other modes and forms of gambling, but appears to be increasing. Few national prevalence studies have been conducted, but international estimates indicate that between 1% and 30% of adults gamble online (Gainsbury 2010; Petry 2006; Wardle et al. 2011b; Wood and Williams 2010). The global Internet gambling market appears to be growing at a rate of approximately 10% per annum, and represents an increasingly important segment of the worldwide gambling industry (Kelleher 2010; Global Betting and Gaming Consultants, GBGC 2010).

The Internet gambling market is being driven by several key trends:

- Fast, cheap broadband access has increased worldwide providing easy access for customers to online betting in addition to access to information on online gambling sites, payment options, sports information, odds and competitive bonuses, and facilitating communication between players. Internet usage and penetration has increased substantially, growing 480% since 2000 worldwide (Miniwatts Marketing Group 2011a). The majority of the population in Europe, North America and Australasia have access to the Internet through computers and mobile phones, and penetration of Internet access has grown over 1,000% in Africa, the Middle East and Latin America and the Caribbean since 2000 (Miniwatts Marketing Group 2011a).
- Liberalised regulation of Internet gambling has increased internationally with growing recognition of the difficulties associated with prohibition, economic benefits of licensing and revenue and the importance of providing player safeguards. Regulated sites may be deemed safer by consumers and provide legitimacy to Internet gambling.
- Televised sport events, both major and minor, has increased visibility with more digital and cable television channels, attracting interest to sports and betting among new audiences.
- Increased consumer confidence in Internet commerce and transactions accompanied by increased security measures providing a greater perception of safety and trust.
- Live products and other innovations are enticing new and existing players as new technologies allow fast-paced, interactive and exciting betting options, including 'exotic' bets and betting on a wider range of sports, games, and events.
- Bingo and 'softer/gaming options', including lotteries and instant/scratch games, are highly appealing to non-traditional gambling markets, particularly women.
- Bonuses and loyalty rewards act to grow the consumer market by encouraging customers to place bets online; however, in the highly competitive market these may be considerable expenses for sites and must be carefully balanced to avoid overextension of budgets.
- New channels for Internet betting include mobile phones and wireless devices (e.g., iPads) are key emerging markets that continue to drive the Internet gambling sector.
- There are an estimated 199 payment methods available for Internet gambling, making it possible for players to make deposits and withdrawals through many channels, avoiding prohibition restrictions. These go beyond Visa, Mastercard and Paypal, all popular payment methods, and include a variety of virtual wallets, prepaid cards, billing systems, wire transfers and payment services.
- Cross-selling of products is now typical as land-based operators and non-gaming companies enter the online market and Internet sites offer a variety of gambling options. Combinations of gambling formats and other products, including social media and gaming, may increase the total number of customers and participation rates.

A highly competitive market now exists based on sophisticated technology and increasingly informed and demanding consumers. The Internet gambling market is characterised by low profit margins and high percentage payouts (Ranade et al. 2006). Estimates for the money going out as winnings range from 88% to 98.7%; the payout percentage is driven by low overhead costs, high customer competition resulting in attractive odds to acquire and retain players, and high turnover ensuing significant profits (Ranade et al. 2006). Reputation and customer trust are very important factors in acquiring and retaining customers, although online gamblers may be fickle displaying little brand loyalty (Church-Sanders 2011; Ranade et al. 2006).

There is clear evidence that Internet gambling participation and revenue are increasing. The rapid growth of Internet gambling has outpaced many of the laws that were created to regulate gambling activities, including models of gambling regulation that concentrate on controlling market entry (through licensing and regulation) and gambling transactions (through surveillance and auditing) (McMillen 2000).

Internet gambling has distinct characteristics that differentiate it from traditional land-based gambling and appeal to new markets. It provides 24-h play, 7 days a week, accessible from almost any location, and games can be fast-paced, continuous, highly interactive, played in a solitary manner, or socially using interactive chat and video features. The nature of the online gambling market is shaped by the regulatory regimes in place, which vary significantly between jurisdictions. Public policy regarding Internet gambling is further complicated by the increasing omnipresence of the Internet, anonymity of users and operators, lack of physical boundaries between jurisdictions, and disparity in physical locations of players and providers. In many cases the legal and regulatory position of Internet gambling is unclear and open to different interpretations, creating uncertainly for customers and operators alike. Due to the relative newness of the Internet gambling phenomenon, there is little historic precedent on which regulators can base policies, and there is certainly no "gold standard" or proven effective policy which has been implemented internationally. Consequentially, many policies and regulations currently in place are ineffective.

Concerns have been expressed about certain features of Internet gambling including the lack of safeguards to prevent minors from gambling, and player protection for problem and pathological gamblers, intoxicated or other vulnerable individuals. There remain considerable difficulties regarding increased affiliations between online gambling operators and sports teams and events, prominent advertisements during games, match-fixing and cheating, fraudulent and unfair play, security and privacy, enforcing regulatory requirements, and provision of responsible play.

Internet gambling remains a reality that must be addressed by governments in a socially responsible manner to help protect and reduce the potential harms associated with excessive use (Monaghan 2009a). As such, it is recommended that key stakeholders carefully examine the many issues surrounding Internet gambling, particularly in terms of the psychosocial impacts, its impact on problem gambling and vulnerable populations and take the necessary steps to implement appropriate policies. The Internet gambling field is characterized by a deficient in research including an understanding of the nature of and participation in online gambling. Internet gambling poses both challenges and opportunities and it is essential that researchers, industry and government act to respond to Internet gambling and the numerous related social issues.

Chapter 2
Current Market Overview

Abstract Internet gambling revenues are predicted to continue to outpace the growth of the global gambling market and represent an increasing proportion of international revenues. Participation and expenditure are increasing despite attempts at restriction and prohibition in several key markets, including the US and China. As much of online gambling is conducted with offshore providers and privately held companies, the size and breakdown of the market can only be estimated. The current chapter outlines the current and predicted revenue and market overview of online gambling, including breakdown by product and region. The prevalence of online gambling is discussed including an overview of available research and estimations of market size. The chapter also outlines each mode of online gambling, including wagering, lotteries, casino games, gaming machines, poker and bingo. Insights are provided into marketing initiatives, payment methods and how customers are acquired and retained. Finally, the key mediums for online gambling, computer, mobile and interactive television are discussed with evidence presented on the current and predicted use of these methods for interactive gambling.

Keywords Mobile gambling • Online gaming • Internet gaming • Revenue • Market share • Regional share • Prevalence • Payment methods • Interactive television

Revenue

Internet gambling revenues (often measured as gross gambling yield; GGY[1]) have increased from approximately US$2.2 billion in 2000 to US$15.2 billion in 2006 and were predicted to reach US$24.5 billion by 2010 (Christiansen Capitol

---

[1] Gross gambling yield or win refers to total amount wagered, less prizes paid to customers. This is a useful measure of how much an online gambling operator earns before taxes, salaries and other expenses such as commission to affiliates, discounted wagers and direct supplier costs are paid. GGY can equal gross profit if there are no other income streams other than gambling.

S. Gainsbury, *Internet Gambling: Current Research Findings and Implications*,
SpringerBriefs in Behavioral Medicine 1, DOI 10.1007/978-1-4614-3390-3_2,
© Springer Science+Business Media, LLC 2012

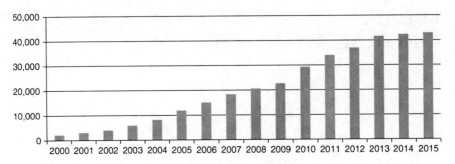

Fig. 2.1 Estimated global Internet gambling yield (US$ million)

Advisors 2005, 2007). More recent reports suggest that the global Internet gambling industry will reach US$33 billion in 2011, despite market setbacks related to the US crackdown on poker and the Japanese earthquake that disrupted the Japanese Racing Association's interactive business (New H2 eGaming dataset now available 2011). This represents around 8% of the entire global gambling market, and with strong underlying growth at 12% global Internet GGY is expected to exceed US$43 billion by 2015 as shown in Fig. 2.1 (GBGC 2011a; Holliday 2010; Holliday 2011; Kelleher 2010; 'New H2 eGaming dataset' 2011).

H2 Gambling Capital qualified their market estimate by stating that the global Internet gambling market available to most operators is actually €13 billion, not €23 billion ('New H2 eGaming dataset' 2011). This adjustment considers the markets and products that are not available to the majority of the listed commercial Internet gambling market, including the Japanese and Hong Kong monopoly betting markets, state lottery markets and the US. The addressable commercial gambling market has still increased, up 52% from 2007 and is expected to increase at a greater rate compared to the total expected sector increase, meaning that the addressable market will account for 62% of the total gambling market in 2011.

Analysts at Juniper Research reported that the online gambling industry is largely recession proof, and growth did occur in this sector during the global financial crisis in the end of the 2000s, perhaps as a result of consumers spending more leisure time at home (iGaming Business 2009). However, evidence from publicly-traded gambling companies showed that online poker revenues decreased in 2009, for example 888 Poker had a 35% reduction to US$26.2 million in the first half of 2009 and Ladbrokes and PartyGaming poker revenue was down 21% and 31% respectively (iGaming Business 2009).

Product Market Share

Industry estimates suggest that betting/wagering (including sports, race, exotic wagering and betting exchanges) leads the global Internet gambling market, accounting for 39% of online gambling (as shown in Fig. 2.2), despite representing

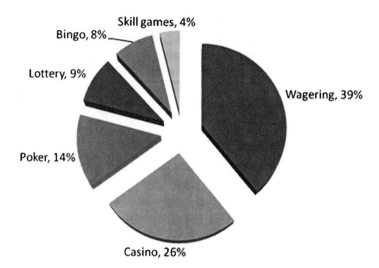

Fig. 2.2 Estimated global Internet gambling market share by product

only 5% of total global gambling GGY ('New H2 eGaming dataset' 2011; Henwood 2011). Reports estimate that the amount bet on online sports betting globally in 2011will reach US$65.1 billion with a gross win of US$5.3 billion (Henwood 2011). The UK, Ireland and Australia appear to be the strongest current markets, although new regulation is opening online markets in Europe, including Spain, Germany, Greece, Denmark and Italy and regulation is being debated in the US (Henwood 2011). In 2010 sports betting was estimated to grow by 12%, primarily driven by the World Cup (Kelleher 2010). UK-based online gambling expert Latitude Digital Marketing predicted a 700% rise in online betting compared to the 2006 tournament and some claimed that over US$5 billion would be spent on the event (Church-Sanders 2011). The online sports betting market is also driven by the increased use of live betting and other product innovations and mobile gambling (Holliday 2010).

Casino games account for 26% of the online gambling market and reflect a strong growth area with slot and other side games increasingly important (Holliday 2010). Casino sites offer increased interactivity and live casinos are seeing strong growth (Holliday 2010).

Online poker now represents just 14%, reduced from 17% in 2006 before the UIGEA prohibited online gambling in the US ('New H2 eGaming dataset' 2011; Holliday 2010). This market faces some uncertainty as the impacts of US prosecutions (detailed in Chap. 3) are still emerging.

Online lotteries are growing (estimated growth 18.6% in 2010) as more and more state lotteries move online and account for 9% of 2011 GGY followed by bingo (approximately 8%) and skill-based and other gaming (approximately 4%; 'New H2 eGaming dataset' 2011; Holliday 2010). However, bingo and other gaming sites are also among the fastest growing market sectors, estimated to grow in 2010 by 21.5% and 18.4% respectively (Holliday 2010). Recent actions by the US Government to prosecute online bingo sites in a similar fashion to online poker sites (Williams 2011) may have an impact on the online bingo market.

Regional Market Share

Europe appears to be the strongest growth market for Internet gambling, representing 47.2% of the global Internet gambling market, up from 31.5% in 2006 ('New H2 eGaming dataset' 2011). Europe is a relatively mature market and growth is being driven by increased liberalisation of regulation and product innovation. The largest European markets include Germany, the UK, Italy and France. The UK is estimated to be the third largest market worldwide accounting for approximately 11% of all online gambling revenue. Following the examples of the UK and Italy, and under pressure from the European Commission, many other countries are currently preparing for a controlled opening of their markets to Internet gambling (KPMG 2010).

North America represented 30.5% of the global market in 2006, before the introduction of UIGEA, which prohibits monetary transfers to online gambling sites; it is expected to be 16.7% in 2011 ('New H2 eGaming dataset' 2011). Prohibition and the recent actions taken by authorities to prosecute offshore Internet gambling sites in the US has reduced the size of this Internet gambling market. The US is still one of the largest worldwide markets, although the full impacts of the recent prosecutions are yet to be seen.

Asia and the Middle East account for 27.7% of the market in 2011, which is 4.5% lower than in 2006 ('New H2 eGaming dataset' 2011). Japan is the single largest Asian market and the second largest market worldwide with 14% of online wagering. Asia is dominated by horse monopolies, such as the Japanese Racing Association, the largest interactive operator in the world, and a small number of commercial sports betting companies (Holliday 2010; 'New H2 eGaming dataset' 2011).

Of the remaining regions, Oceania and Australia hold approximately 5% of the market, leaving Central and South America and the Caribbean with 3% and Africa with 1% (Holliday 2010).

KPMG consulting firm reported that market growth is based on the key factors of solid broadband Internet infrastructure and penetration, easy access to mobile applications, and safe and secure payments through a native banking system (KPMG 2010). They estimate that key emerging regions to be targeted by operators include India and Latin America (Fig. 2.3).

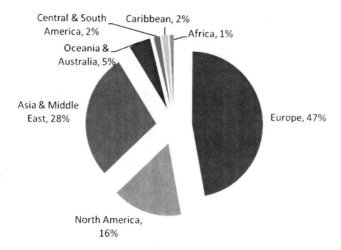

Fig. 2.3 Regional Internet gambling market share

Prevalence

Technological developments and policy changes have resulted in high-speed, low-cost Internet facilities accessible globally; 77% usage in North American, 80% Australian and New Zealand, 71% UK, 58–86% European, 34% Latin America, 30% Middle East, 22% Asia, 11% Africa, and 24% world-wide, respectively (Miniwatts Marketing Group 2010). Although heavily used by individuals under the age of 34, middle-age and older adults are increasingly accessing the Internet daily; for example, in Canada 83% of 16–34 year-olds, followed by 72% of 35–54, 69% of 55–64, and 66% of 65+ year-olds, with these rates increasing annually (Statistics Canada 2010). High quality and high speed Internet access and associated technologies (computers, smart-phones, iPad and webcams) are not only becoming more affordable but also accessible through computers located in educational institutes, cafes and public libraries (Phillips and Blaszczynski 2010).

Estimates of the prevalence of Internet gambling participation are limited as few conclusive studies have been conducted internationally. Many studies examining Internet gambling use small, non-representative samples limiting the extent to which results can be generalised to the general population. Prevalence rates that have been reported are based on disparate methodologies making comparisons difficult. Many jurisdictions do not have accurate estimates and prevalence studies, when conducted, may include Internet gambling under 'other' forms of gambling. The validity of prevalence surveys has been questioned, for example, Warwick Bartlett of GBGC claims that the illegal nature of Internet gambling in many jurisdictions may result

Table 2.1 Estimated international Internet gambling prevalence – country comparisons

Country	Prevalence	Reference
Australia	1–4.3%	Productivity Commission (2010)
New Zealand	2%	Gray (2011)
Singapore	1%	Ministry of Community Development, Youth and Sports (2008)
China	2%	Stradbrooke (2011)
South Korea	4.3%	Park et al. (2010)
Hungary	1.3%	Kun et al. (2011)
United Kingdom	13%	Wardle et al. (2011b)
Northern Ireland	3.2%	Department for Social Development (2010)
Iceland	1.6%	Olason (2009)
Finland	13%	Olason (2009)
Norway	6.5%	Sandven (2007)
Sweden	9%	Swedish National Institute of Public Health (2011)
Denmark	10.8%	Bonke (2007)
Germany	2.2%	Bundeszentrale für gesundheitliche Aufklärung (2010)
Netherlands	3.5%	Motivation (2005)
Canada	2–8%	Ipsos Reid (2010); Wood and Williams (2010)
Spain	2.4%	Volberg (2010)
United States	2–7%	American Gaming Association (2010); Petry (2006)

Notes:
1. Different estimates for an individual country represent disparity in reported prevalence rates
2. Studies utilised different methodology so comparisons must be treated with caution
3. Rapid changes in Internet gambling result in some prevalence figures becoming quickly outdated

in underestimates of the actual gambling market, making participation figures appear inflated in regulated, legalised markets, such as the UK ('Gambling commission prevalence survey flawed' 2011). Table 2.1 shows the results of Internet gambling prevalence studies that have been reported. It is important to note that the rapid growth of Internet gambling means that older findings may be outdated.

Customer Acquisition and Retention

Player acquisition and retention is a crucial element of a successful online gambling site, which requires sites to understand and cater for customers in addition to traditional marketing efforts for new and existing players (Church-Sanders 2011). Industry reports indicated that in 2009 online gambling operators were required to spend around US$30,000–$50,000 monthly on marketing if they were to be able to complete with the established brands or those with more money to spend on bonuses (iGaming Business 2009). Some online gambling operators reportedly to spend over US$1 million per month on marketing alone (iGaming Business 2009). In the first half of 2010 there were steep increases in marketing spend following the recession, and to coincide with the 2010 FIFA World Cup; Bwin increased its spend by 30%, 888 by 20% and Paddy Power by 50% (Church-Sanders 2011).

Many Internet gambling sites offer signup bonuses to new players, which usually require a minimum amount of wagering before allowing a cash-out. Bonuses may also be offered for player loyalty, repeat deposits and referring a friend including bonus credits/money, matching a certain proportion of deposits (e.g., 10%), free spins on particular games and play for a predetermined period of time with a set amount of dollars. Players must open an account with the site, which is generally facilitated with a credit or debit card, or through direct money or bank wire transfers.

To be viable, operators must develop strategies to differentiate themselves from other sites and retain a competitive advantage through creation of positive and preferential customer attitudes and repeat gambling patronage. User confidence, trust in regulators and operators, payment processing problems and regulation all pose constraints to the growth and success of Internet gambling (Dinev et al. 2006; McCole et al. 2010; Paul Budd Communication 2010). Research indicates that the key factors which influence Internet gambling behavior include player satisfaction, customer service, security and privacy, website reliability and third party endorsement (Chen 2005; Gainsbury et al. unpublished manuscript; Guo et al. 2009; Jolley et al. 2006; McCole et al. 2010; Woolley 2003). Online gamblers want a fast, reliable, clear and intuitive experience and if they experience difficulties they are likely to give up quickly and turn to another site (Church-Sanders 2011).

Internet gambling operators need to make customers feel safe and secure. Security concerns, trust in payment systems and legitimacy appear to be primary reasons for not playing online (Ipsos Reid 2005; Woodruff and Gregory 2005). Internet gamblers also have significant concerns with fair play practices and cheating (Wood and Griffiths 2008; Wood and Williams 2010). A study by the American Gaming Association (AGA 2006) shows that 55% of a sample of online gamblers believe that online casinos cheat players and 46% believe that players have found a way to cheat the sites. A UK study found that consumers feel gambling websites fail to provide appropriate levels of customer support and that upwards of 92% of gambling websites fail to provide sufficient information and contacts details (Talisma 2007). Player concerns are not unfounded, as described in a later chapter, there are numerous examples of online gambling sites going bankrupt, not paying winnings or deposits, cheating players with unfair games and failing to protect personal information (Games and Casino 2006; McMullan and Rege 2010).

An online survey of a large sample of international gamblers (N = 12,521) investigated the main reasons Internet gamblers prefer one gambling site over another (Wood and Williams 2010). The general reputation of the site was the most commonly reported reason (18%), reflecting the importance of branding. Customer experience is also very important with 12% of participants citing better game experience and interface of a particular gambling site, making this the second most common factor. Comps and bonuses were important factors for 10% of participants and payout rates were cited by 8% of participants as the reason they choose a particular gambling site. Security and trust appear to be key concerns as monetary deposits being safe and wins paid out in a timely fashion were important to 10% of players and fairness of games reported by 9%. Legality and operating jurisdiction were cited by only 6% and 3% of participants respectively, indicating that many players are not aware of these factors, or not highly influenced by them.

These results are somewhat similar to results found by eCOGRA (e-Commerce and Online Gaming Regulation and Assurance), which reported that bonuses (75%), followed by game variety (62%), deposit method and reputation (both 56%) and promptness of payouts (54%) were the most important factors in choosing a site (Church-Sanders 2011).

Payment Methods

Players can use a variety of payment options to make deposits and withdrawals from online gambling sites. According to Casino City there are over 199 different payment methods available for online gambling sites. The most common payment methods for online gambling sites are credit cards and debit cards, used by the vast majority of players, followed by eWallets, bank and monetary transfer systems, and prepaid cards (European Commission 2011a; iGaming Business 2009). Visa and Mastercard are the most popular payment method, accepted by 91% and 87% of Internet gambling sites respectively, although restrictions block US players (Casino City Online 2011). Other popular methods made available to players include Neteller (72% of sites), Moneybookers, a virtual wallet (68%), Bank Wire Transfer (65%), or Maestro, a debit card from Mastercard (45%).

Credit cards are different from debit cards as they do not remove money from the user's account after each transaction and do not require full payment each month. Rather, credit cards lend money to consumers, similar to a cash advance, and allow customers to pay the balance when they are able, with interest rates applied. Paying with credit cards online is generally considered safe as most reputable gambling sites use high levels of security to encrypt payment information and protect customers. Credit cards many also reimburse customers if they are victims of fraud. It is important for customers to realise that payments to online sites are typically identified as cash advances, and as such have higher fees and interest rates applied. Individuals using credit cards to pay for online gambling should be careful to avoid making more transactions than they can afford as interest rates can result in high levels of debts.

Debit cards are similar to credit cards, however their functionality is like writing a cheque as funds are directly withdrawn from customer's bank accounts. Payment through this method is taken and verified after each transaction (typically through PIN codes) with debits immediately registered in accounts. The card issuer has to approve transactions in order to ensure that funds are available, which makes it more difficult to use this method of payment in jurisdictions that prohibit online gambling.

Internet payment systems or eWallets, such as Equifax, Moneybooker, FirePay, and ClickandBuy and NETeller, serve as a wallet for online purchases and are easy to register for and set up. This is a relatively safe form of payment as the online gambling operator does not have access to an individual's bank or credit card information.

Online payment systems typically require identity verification before customers can use these services, which minimises fraud and prevents money laundering EWallets provide digital cash systems that are easy to use, secure and fast and banks have no way of identifying what the funds were originally used for as the transaction is listed as the online payment system. Some online payment systems, notably PayPal, do not accept gambling-related transactions in jurisdictions where this is not permitted. Given the increased use of the Internet to purchase many items, such as song and movie downloads, online payment systems are becoming more sophisticated and easy to use.

A wire transfer is an electronic bank transfer from one bank to another. These can be done online of through retail outlets and do not require a credit card. One of the largest companies offering this service is Western Union, which has 100,000 agencies worldwide. Some online gambling sites accept cheques send through regular mail, although this is generally very slow. Postal or Money Orders are similar although usually involve going to a bank to pay with cash.

Some regulatory policies make it more difficult to negotiate payment for online gambling sites, notably in the US where the Unlawful Internet Gambling Enforcement Act of 2006 (UIGEA) prohibits financial institutions from processing payments to online gambling sites. Although it is relatively easy for established customers to find ways around these policies, new players may have more difficulties and may choose not to play online as a result (iGaming Business 2009).

There are numerous alternatives to using direct bank transfers or credit card payments that are identifiable as online gambling transactions. Pre-paid credit cards, such as PaySafeCard, Ukash and Entropay, allow users to load cards with credit online, at retail outlets, over the phone or through ATMs, and use the funds to pay for online gambling. Some companies, such as Entropay, allow users to provide payment details and identification as they would any other credit card, so that these cards are acceptable as a form of payment even for sites that demand rigorous customer identification.

Types of Internet Gambling Sites

There are several business models of Internet gambling sites in addition to the range of products offered. Some sites are able to achieve liquidity[2] independently, whereas others generate traffic through membership of a larger network and sharing software and promotions. Standalone sites are powered by propriety software that is not used by any other gambling site (Church-Sanders 2011). These sites do not share offerings or chatrooms, own their own data and usually have their own support teams. Another model is for sites to license software from an independent developer, which provides software to other sites (Church-Sanders 2011). Typically these

---

[2] Liquidity refers to the volume of active customers that online gambling platforms need to be able to offer them a wide variety of games or betting markets

sites have unique promotions and offers, including the types of gambling options offered. Software companies typically earn a share of the revenue from sites that use their products. Stand alone and licensing models offer greater independence and flexibility as well as control of campaigns and bonuses, and a propriety database. Standalone models also have no network limitations and unique games and products, whilst licensed sites save costs on software and have access to a wide range of products and games.

Some smaller sites may be serviced by one operator or software company and have their own 'front end' owners within the operation, colloquially referred to as 'skins' (Church-Sanders 2011). Such a network of sites may comprise of two or more sites that are affiliated with each other and share the same software, but are typically managed individually. Being part of a network allows a skin owner to use the products and chatrooms as well as technicians and support provided by the operator while being responsible for advertising, promotions and affiliates. Network owners receive a proportion of all bets placed with their operation from the various skins connected in addition to an upfront fee and proportion of gross operating profits. Networks are more common for poker, casino, bingo and skill games than sportsbook sites. They have advantages in terms of low barrier to enter the market, instant liquidity, product knowledge and marketing expertise, minimal infrastructure costs and ability to bring a brand to the market quickly.

Online Casino Games

Online casinos were among the first gaming sites to appear on the Internet when launched in the mid-1990s (Church-Sanders 2010). Online casino games remain a leading gaming genre, comprising approximately 33% of market sites in 2010 (ZagZig Media Analysis reported by Church-Sanders 2010). Typical online casino games include Slot machines and video poker games, Blackjack, Poker variations, Craps, Roulette, Baccarat, Let' em ride, Virtual racing, and Pai Gow Poker. Technological innovations have resulted in an increasingly sophisticated array of games, many of which closely replicate land-based gaming although others now incorporate video-clips and a broader entertainment value (Church-Sanders 2010). Customers may be required to download software to play games, which benefits players as downloaded games typically run faster than those played directly from the site after the initial set-up time.

Online casinos generally offer odds and payback percentages that are comparable to or better than land-based casinos with random number generators used to ensure that the numbers, cards or dice appear randomly. Casino table games have more favourable returns with a loss rate of 2.3%. Player payback percentage or return to player can be greater at online casinos as these are much cheaper to start-up and run than land-based venues, costing on average US$1.5 million at start-up with few employees required (Church-Sanders 2010). Many sites publish the odds of winning on different games, for example, bwin Interactive Entertainment lists video poker and slots as having the lowest player returns; overall losses of 6.2% and 5.8% respectively (https://casino.bwin.com/casino.aspx?view=payoutTable). Games with short playing times, such as slots, appear to generate the majority of money for online casino providers as more games can be played per unit of time (Church-Sanders 2010).

The online casino gaming industry is characterised by networks, software companies and standalone operators and include sites that exclusively offer casino games, or those that have added casino games to their existing portfolio of online gambling products (Church-Sanders 2010). Entertainment is an important element of customer satisfaction and new games with a variety of skill levels must be constantly offered to retain players (Church-Sanders 2010). The speed at which new games can be introduced into the market enables online casinos to capitalise on trends and offer products that have a broad appeal and are easy to learn and play, which may account for their large market share. For example, in February 2010, winter sports-themed slot machines were launched and promoted to coincide with the Vancouver Winter Olympics.

According to a large scale survey of Internet gamblers (eCOGRA 2007), the typical Internet casino player was likely to be female (55%), between 46 and 55 years of age (30%), playing 2–3 times per week (37%), playing between 1 and 2 h per session (27%), and wagering between $30 and $60 per session (18%). The survey further revealed that the most important concerns held by online casino game players focused upon financial or security issues; including good bonus promotions, deposit methods and a solid reputation. Additionally, participants wanted sites to include multiple games. Motivations reported for gambling on these Internet casino sites included participating for relaxation, excitement, distraction, opportunities to make money, and escape. Gambling for social reasons was not a predominant motivation. Those who tended to lose more money were individuals gambling for excitement, to relieve boredom and as a way to facilitate escaping problems.

Online Poker

Online poker is one of the most popular forms of online gambling, constituting approximately 19% of the global Internet gambling market (Holliday 2010). Online poker rooms allow players to play for stakes as low as one cent. Many sites offer free poker, where no real money is wagered, although in some cases players can accumulate credits that can be exchanged for prizes. Free poker sites are often marketed as instructional sites for inexperienced players to allow them to gain confidence and learn some basic skills. Free poker sites typically require players to be registered and have an account and often have no age limits.

Real money Internet poker generated rakes/tournament fees of US$4.91 billion in 2009, up 28% from 2010 (Holliday 2010). Industry reports indicate that the vast majority of play is at micro stakes games; the average pot size is US$11.44 and the average prize paying tournament buy in is US$1.65 (Holliday 2010). The average number of real money players seated per table is 5.4, with an average of 21,350 tables open and 115,000 players online (Holliday 2010). Online poker is more popular in the evening as the peak period for all major sites is 18:00 to 24:00 BST (Holliday 2010).

Standalone poker sites and poker networks represent a minority of poker sites as the vast majority of online poker sites are independent doorways or 'skins' into the group of network sites (iGaming Business 2009). However, the majority of online poker traffic occurs on just a few major networks including Party Poker, PokerStars, Full Tilt Poker, 888poker and the iPoker Network (iGaming Business 2009). Online poker operators must be able to successfully attract and retain players and to ensure that they have sufficient liquidity so that players are always able to find a range of games at various levels of skill and price.

In addition to the factors that have driven the Internet gambling market in general, the growth in the poker industry is linked to:

- Increased television exposure
- Reciprocal movement between online and land-based poker-play
- Celebrity participation
- High publicity for winners, including previously unknown players who won entry through online play
- High net-worth prizes, including entry to tournaments
- Relatively low barriers to entry
- Tools to assist beginners including free play sites and instructions (iGaming Business 2009).

In April 2011 US authorities took actions to prosecute several large poker sites that are accused of numerous legal breaches, which is described in more detail in relation to US Internet gambling policy in Chap. 3. This has decimated the scale of the Internet poker industry in the US (Holliday 2010). At this stage it is calculated that the impact will equate to as much as USD$1,076 million of lost market value in 2011 and a further USD$140 million loss in 2012 ('New H2 eGaming dataset' 2011). Player volume from April 14 to April 25 for Full Tilt Poker declined 36.8% and PokerStars declined 15.9%, with losses still sustained in May 2011 (Holliday 2010). Prior to the April indictments, it was estimated that 2.5 million people played online poker in the US, this has been reduced to a small fraction (Vardi 2011). Industry reports indicate that Internet poker will still glow globally in 2011/12, but that at least half of the US market may be lost, although it is difficult to forecast the exact impact and the policy changes to come (Holliday 2010).

There is ongoing debate over whether poker should be classified as a game of chance or skill. A game of skill is characterised by the outcome of a game being predominately influenced by skill elements rather than chance (Fiedler and Rock 2009). The parameters of legal poker playing are still unclear and differ between jurisdictions (Grohman 2006; Kelly et al. 2007). In poker, a player has several options for actions that will influence the outcome of the game (folding, calling, betting, raising, and re-raising). Interpreting and weighing the influencing factors and correctly making a decision and acting out the strategy requires skill. However, it is difficult to isolate and measure all the skill elements to determine their contribution to the outcome. Several jurisdictions have found that skill is a significant component in the game and plays a role in determining the outcome (Fiedler and Rock 2009), which has considerable impact on subsequent policies and regulations. In an influential paper, Dreef et al. (cited by Fiedler and Rock 2009) emphasised that the element of skill in poker is relative to the skill of the other players and the magnitude of chance elements. Despite the element of skill involved, poker is still considered a game of chance, hence a gambling activity. Although in the long run, skill might predominate over chance, particularly for more experienced players, for each individual session or over a short period of time (months to a year), the outcome of poker is determined by chance (Grohman 2006). For example, a skilled player may know that his poker-hand has an 85% chance of beating his opponent's hand, but 15% of the time, the player will lose the hand and the money staked.

Aside from the argument of the role of skill, proponents of online poker have claimed that since the operators of poker sites only take a proportion of the amount bet (a rake) so do not play against patrons or have a stake in the outcome of any game, that they should not be considered as gambling operators ('Defence in NYC prosecution' 2011). However, from a political perspective, regulating gambling is typically based on the potential for social costs and online poker, as with other forms of online gambling, can result in significant negative consequences for individuals (Bjerg 2010; Gainsbury 2010).

There are substantial differences between online poker gaming and conventional in-person gaming. One obvious difference is that players cannot see each other resulting in players using different means to attempt to predict player behaviour including betting patterns, reaction time, speed of play, etc. As online poker is not delayed by shuffling and dealing cards, the rate of play is much faster than in an actual game and depending on the site a player might play several tables simultaneously. Even playing at a single table of six players in a land-based venue, a player can expect to play approximately 30 hands an hour, compared with 75 hands per hour at an online casino (Fiedler and Rock 2009). Online players typically play 4–6, or even 12–16, tables simultaneously (Fiedler and Rock 2009). Poker tournaments require a certain commitment from players in terms of time and money staked, while cash or ring games allow players to join and leave at any time (iGaming Business 2009).

The most common age group for poker players is between 18 and 35, and is more popular among males (at a ratio of around 85/15) (eCOGRA 2007; iGaming Business 2009). In general, younger players appear to be more successful and stronger players than other age cohorts (iGaming Business 2009). In a survey of Internet gamblers, eCOGRA (2007) reported the typical online poker player played 2–3 times per week (27%), have played for 2–3 years (24%), played between 1 and 2 h per session (33%), played one (24%) or two (24%) tables simultaneously, and played at minimum stake levels of $0.50–$2.00 (61%). Sites allow players to customise the look and feel of their playing environment and choose avatars and screen names to represent themselves. Some research indicates that players may swap genders when playing online (Wood et al. 2007).

Online Sports Betting

Increasing sophistication and options of wagers allow gamblers to bet on almost any aspect of an event. Sports betting is distinct from other forms of online gambling in that customers may primarily be involved with another activity, that is, watching sports, rather than the gambling being the entertainment activity itself (Church-Sanders 2011). This may vary, as some customers are superstitious and will force themselves not to watch games on which they have bet (Church-Sanders 2011).

The online sports betting market has been driven by increased availability of televised events, including amateur, youth and college events in a wide range of sports. The Internet also provides access to a wealth of information enabling customers to be highly informed, which may increase the perception that one is betting strategically. Blogs, chatrooms, forums and other sites also provide easy access to tips, best odds and bonuses and predictions to assist new players in placing bets online. Online betting operators are also offering a range of mobile applications, live betting, side casino or poker games, exotic betting options and video streaming making Internet betting more attractive and entertaining (Church-Sanders 2011).

There are several variants of betting offered online:

- Fixed odds betting is the most popular form of sports betting, both online and offline, in which the bookmaker offers odds for sports events (Church-Sanders 2011). Common fixed odds bets include the win bet, each-way bet and place bet. Exotic bets are bets on outcomes within the game for example, who makes the opening goal, the score at the first half, etc.
- Spread betting is increasingly popular and requires accuracy rather than predicting the outcomes of an event (Church-Sanders 2011). The bookmaker gives an advantage to the weaker team and the customer bets on whether the actual outcome will be higher or lower than the sportsbook's prediction. Wins are determined by the difference between the operator's prediction and the actual result and the wager made.
- In live-action betting, or in-play gambling bets are made on real time propositions about outcomes within a sporting event. In-play betting may also refer to placing wagers on the outcome of an event after that event has started. Live betting has grown in popularity and now accounts for 40–50% of bets for some online players (Church-Sanders 2011). Some sports betting operators claim that live-action betting accounts for 30–70% of gross margins (Church-Sanders 2011). Types of live-action bets include which team will score next, whether a play will be completed, penalties given, etc. Live-action betting may be riskier than fixed-odds betting and may be more associated with gambling-related problems (LaPlante et al. 2008). This may be due to the high number of bets that can be placed during a single event.
- Parimutuel betting is a system where customers place their bets in a pool and after the outcome of an event is known, the payout odds are calculated and the winnings are distributed among all the winning bets, minus the fee to the operator (Church-Sanders 2011).

Betting Exchanges

Betting exchanges are sites that are growing in popularity by creating a marketplace for bettors where potential wagers are posted on certain events (with accompanying odds and stake size) which individuals may accept (Koning and van Velzen 2009). Although these wagers primarily focus on sporting and racing events, they also include wagers ranging from the outcome of political elections, events on reality television, wagering on winners of music or dance contests, and outrageous behaviour of popular celebrities (Koning and van Velzen 2009).

Betting exchanges are attractive as they allow players to create their own odds, typically offer better odds than traditional bookmakers and have a lower operator take (Church-Sanders 2011). Players can also 'lay' selection, which means predicting outcomes that will not happen, a function that can also be used by bettors to adjust their betting position at a later time by buying or selling back bets at different odds, theoretically allowing an individual to make a profit before the event has even stated. Betting exchanges have low operating risks as they are not a party in any betting transaction and make money regardless of the outcome of the event (Koning and van Velzen 2009). As betting exchanges do not have to set odds, this lowers operational costs related to obtaining information, monitoring events and creating markets. However, to be profitable, betting exchanges must have sufficient liquidity (active customers) to be able to attract new users. Bookmakers also may offer loyalty bonuses and certain percentage guarantees to large bettors, which may restrict the potential market for betting exchanges.

The largest betting exchange is Betfair, which reportedly has five million transactions a day, comprising 90% of the betting exchange market and more than all the stock exchanges in Europe (Church-Sanders 2011). Betfair charges a commission of 5% on each winning bet and commissions are lowered as players bet more.

Online Bingo

Bingo is one of the most popular and socially accepted games in the world with industry figures conservatively indicating that over 100 million people play the game in land-based locations (Screen Digest 2009). Online bingo is similar to online casino games with sites using random number generators to draw virtual balls. Many sites offer multiple forms of bingo with different features, types of games and costs of play. Bingo sites commonly feature a chat application which encourages players to chat with each other, attempting to create a friendly and communal atmosphere and functioning as an effective retention tool (KPMG 2010). These sites often cater specifically for women and some research suggests that they may appeal to markets who would not typically engage in traditional forms of gambling (Corney and Davis 2010; Wood, Williams, and Lawton 2007). This is consistent with the perception that bingo is a safe pastime, played by people who would not typically engage in other gambling activities such as casino gambling or betting (Screen Digest 2009).

According to a study by media analyst Screen Digest (2009), with growing broadband penetration, increased promotions, a trend towards regulatory relaxation and current economic downturn driving demand for in-home entertainment, online bingo has become the fastest growing sector of the online gambling market and has huge potential for future growth. The UK market is well established and was estimated to generate over €220 million of revenue in 2008 (gross win) (Screen Digest 2009). Potential markets for expansion of online bingo include Spain, and select markets in Eastern Europe, Asia and Latin America (Screen Digest 2009).

Online Lotteries

Online lotteries were the first and one of the most popular forms of gambling to capitalize on the use of the Internet. Online lottery sites allow gamblers to participate in state, provincial or international lotteries (this varies depending upon the jurisdiction and the site offering these services) via online purchase of tickets. These sites also provide the results for international lotteries. As more jurisdictions begin regulating Internet gambling, online lotteries are being increasingly operated by state and provincial government bodies, with some offering land-based lottery draws, or the opportunity to purchase tickets on a regular basis (particularly appealing for individuals who play the same numbers weekly) for land-based draws using the Internet rather than having to physically purchase a ticket from a vendor. Online lotteries, such as those offered in Canada and the UK, have been developed as a way of creating new opportunities for existing players and attract new customers as well as increasing revenues. Within the US, this method of offering lottery tickets is perceived to not only help in sustaining revenue but is perceived as one of the most important ways of growing a player-base over time (Jackson 2008). Online instant scratch tickets are also available online. Industry reports estimate that mobile lotteries will account for 41% of total mobile gambling expenditure in the next 5 years (Paul Budd Communication 2010).

Skill Gaming Sites

Skill game sites offer a wide diversity of games including work games, puzzles, strategy games (e.g., mahjong, chess), sports (e.g., billiards, golf, racing), cards, arcade, trivia and videogames (Wood and Williams 2007). Skill games differ from traditional casino games, such as bingo or poker as they are not considered "games of chance" given the outcome of a game is dependent upon the player's skill and/or knowledge of a specific contest or subject. As such, these sites are considered legal in certain jurisdictions that ban Internet gambling. These sites typically offer tournaments whereby a player pays a fee to enter and the winner collects a prize in addition to single-player and per-game wagers.

Practice Sites

In addition to the various forms of Internet gambling activities, many site also offer "practice" or "free play" games where customers can engage in gambling-type games without wagering real money or depositing funds into an account. Typically, these games have no age restrictions. These sites are often marketed as instructional sites to assist players to learn the rules and procedures associated with the particular gambling activity and they are often linked to real money sites or games. Although commercials stress the fun and 'educational' nature of the sites, they have been referred as a "Trojan Horse" strategy used by online gambling companies to acquire players who will eventually transfer to the 'real-money' gambling sites (Monaghan and Derevensky 2008). Online gamblers may use money sites and free plays sites, for example, in a survey of 563 online gamblers, 42% of respondents reported having gambled online in the past year and 77% had played on practice, or free sites (McBride and Derevensky 2009). The most common reasons provided for playing on practice sites included fun, entertainment, relaxation, to relieve boredom, and excitement.

Modes of Interactive Gambling

The vast majority of online gambling is conducted through personal computers connected to the Internet. Computers provide large screens (multiple screens can be used simultaneously) and fast processors to enable sites to provide sophisticated graphics and technology. However, technological improvements and increased penetration of other Internet-enabled devices is changing the way in which customers are experiencing Internet gambling. Subsequently, online operators are developing gambling opportunities for new platforms.

Mobile Gambling

Mobile gambling refers to gambling undertaken on a remote wirelessly connected device. Early versions of mobile gambling services involved subscribers receiving SMS text alerts for lottery results or horse racing odds, which was followed by the launch of the SMS-based betting services that allowed gamblers to bet on horse races. The emergence of sophisticated handsets and advanced mobile data services allowed users to download Java-based gambling applications over high-speed wireless networks with video capabilities. Although traditional websites can generally be accessed through mobile phones connected to the Internet, due to the small screen and keyboards of mobiles, sites and apps have been increasingly adapted for specific use of mobile handsets (Owens 2010). Tablets may also be used for mobile gambling, although they are not as portable as mobile and smart phones, as they have larger screens which may be more suitable for gambling, particularly for longer sessions. Betting dominates the mobile gambling market, due to the ease at which this type of gambling can be adapted to these devices and demand for betting at a range of venues other than the home. However, gaming, including bingo and slot machines, and lotteries, are likely to increasingly be used for mobile gambling.

The global mobile gambling market was valued at US$2.8 billion in 2010, the vast majority of which was accounted for by mobile betting (GBGC 2011b; H2 Gambling Capital 2011). At the end of 2010 the mobile gambling market accounted for 9.8% of interactive and 0.6% of global gambling GGY (H2 Gambling Capital 2011). The largest mobile gambling markets are Japan (race wagering), Hong Kong (race wagering), and the UK (casino and betting) (H2 Gambling Capital 2011; Juniper Research 2010). Europe represents 27% of the entire global market, and outside the UK, key markets include Italy, France, Germany (sports betting only), and Scandinavia (H2 Gambling Capital 2011). The Asian market is over three times larger than Europe; in 2010 the Japanese Racing Association was estimated to account for almost 57% of the value of the global mobile gambling market, although this contribution is expected to be as low as 40% in 2011 following the earthquake and strong growth of mobile gambling in other markets (H2 Gambling Capital 2011). Mobile lottery in China is predicted to grow so that China also will represent a significant market (H2 Gambling Capital 2011; Juniper Research 2010). Several US states are also exploring the introduction of mobile lotteries, as are other juris-dictions, such as New Zealand (Juniper Research 2010; 'New Zealand' 2011). The prevalence of mobile gambling is still relatively low. For example, statistics released by the UK Gambling Commission in August 2011 indicate that 3.2% of respondents reported gambling using mobile phones, up from 2.2% in 2006 (Johan 2011). Australian market research suggests that 2.6% of adults report typically pur-chasing lottery tickets over the Internet (Roy Morgan Research 2010).

Interactive Television

Interactive television was launched in the late 1990s and featured content such as movies on demand. This mode has expanded to include shopping, banking, music, video games, competitions and gambling (Phillips and Blaszczynski 2010). Gambling through interactive television can take multiple forms including directly gambling on sporting events such a horse racing and football using a television remote control, or placing bets on casino games, playing bingo, or purchasing lottery tickets. Questions remain over the classification of games in which players phone a premium-rate telephone line to place a bet or participate in a skill-game such as puzzles, word games and trivia questions.

Interactive television lends itself most obviously to wagering and channels can be offered to digital subscribers, typically run in conjunction with racing and sports channels. Betting services can tell viewers when the next event will be aired and what betting opportunities are available. Multiple gambling opportunities are available, including betting on various events and markets, in a relatively simple format. Gambling products can also be integrated into betting on television shows or virtual racing and sports games as well as offering lotteries, bingo, poker and casino games.

Prevalence data from the UK indicates that only 1.4% of respondents placed bets using interactive or digital television gambling accounts for (Johan 2011). In Australia, Tab Active Interactive TV is the fastest-growing wagering channel of the gambling company Tabcorp (Reichel 2010). In the first year after its launch in April 2008, more than 22,400 users placed at least one bet, turnover exceeded AUD$81 million and 3,000 users were betting each week. In 2010 Tab Active was only available in Sydney and Melbourne, but it was already generating around 2% of Tabcorp's remote betting turnover. At the end of June 2011 total turnover had exceeded AUD$141 million and 16 million bets in total had been placed through the service with an average number of 16.060 bets per day (Twoway Interactive Entertainment 2011). In France, Pari Mutuel Urbain (PMU, the French totaliser monopoly) reported its interactive TV wagering service had five times the turnover of PMU mobile in 2008 (€31.7 million), accounting for 4.3% of total remote betting turnover (Reichel 2010).

Gaming Consoles

Many recently released forms of video gaming consoles allow users to connect to the Internet, which provides further opportunities for interactive gambling. Connecting gaming consoles to the Internet has moved betting on video games from between friends in a lounge room to making wagers between people all over the world. Video betting sites allows players with almost any gaming console to create, enter and bet on tournaments for almost any video game such as the popular Call of Duty and Madden NFL games. The betting site acts as an intermediary, organising the tournaments, collecting the stakes and distributing the final prize to the winner. The amount of money the players may win is dependent on the number of players involved. Gaming consoles are monitored by the site in an effort to prevent players from cheating.

Recent developments in this market include the announcement in 2011 by Virgin Gaming of a deal with Electronic Arts to support a majority of popular sports games, including FIFA Soccer, NHL Hockey, NCAA Fotball, Madden NFL Football and Tiger Woods PGA Tour, using its online wagering system (Pilieci 2011). Virgin allows video gamers to wager on the outcome of their video game challenges and then tracks the players as they play on an Xbox 360 or PS3, ensuring that no one is cheating. The winner is paid up to tens of thousands of dollars. In January, 2011, Virgin Gaming reported that it has 170,000 users from 30 countries signed up to use its online service. At time of press, the Virgin system only allows organised tournaments, meaning players can buy into a tournament and then play for the ultimate win, although developments will allow for game-by-game wagering, allowing gamers to create their own tournaments and challenge others for cash prizes.

Chapter 3
Policy and Regulatory Options

Abstract Multiple regulatory options are currently in place in response to Internet gambling. However, there is currently no "gold standard" or even policies that appear to be highly effective and broadly suitable. This chapter considers the advantages and disadvantages of various policy options, including prohibition, licensing and regulation, as well as restrictions on the sites available, and third party regulation. Specific jurisdictional responses are outlined for many international jurisdictions, including the impact of these on the online gambling market to describe the current policy and regulatory arrangements and any significant issues. This chapter is based on empirical evidence collected from academic and industry research as well as analysis of outcomes and consequences of policy options. Associated issues are discussed including how to uphold and enforce regulations, which is particularly difficult given the global and somewhat anonymous nature of online gambling. The social costs of online gambling are also discussed as well as taxation rates and the impact on other industries, including land-based gambling.

Keywords Policy • Regulation • International • Internet gambling • Online Gaming • North America • Asia Pacific • Europe • Africa • Social Costs • Tax

There is a great deal of confusion amongst regulators, politicians, operators, players and the general public regarding the legality of Internet gambling. The rapid growth of Internet gambling has outpaced many of the laws that were created to regulate gambling activities. Public policy regarding Internet gambling is complicated by the increasing omnipresence of the Internet, anonymity of users and operators, lack of physical boundaries between jurisdictions, and disparity in physical locations of players and providers. Regulation varies widely between countries and even within states and provinces and changes regularly, making it difficult for stakeholders to always fully comprehend legal policies. Some gambling operators claim to spend over £1 million annually on legal advice and fees alone, making this a substantial cost for operators (iGaming Business 2009).

S. Gainsbury, *Internet Gambling: Current Research Findings and Implications*,
SpringerBriefs in Behavioral Medicine 1, DOI 10.1007/978-1-4614-3390-3_3,
© Springer Science+Business Media, LLC 2012

Several jurisdictions have not enacted any specific Internet gambling policies and instead have adapted existing gambling regulations. This causes further confusion amongst operators, consumers and even regulators over the interpretation of gambling laws. For example, the Canadian Criminal Code, which regulates other forms of gambling, does not specifically refer to Internet gambling, but states that the provincial government may operate a lottery. This has been interpreted to allow provincially-owned and operated online gambling sites, including lottery, poker, casino and sports betting (Gainsbury and Wood 2011). New Zealand also has no specific Internet gambling policies, yet the Lotteries Commission is proposing to introduce the sale of online scratch tickets in an attempt to better meet sales quotas ('New Zealand' 2011). It is important for governments and policy makers to carefully consider the unique challenges related to Internet gambling and as far as possible enact appropriate and effective regulations (Gainsbury 2010).

There is currently a large gap in the literature regarding the effectiveness of the different models of regulation. Several jurisdictions, including Australia and the European Union (EU) are currently conducting reviews in an effort to inform regulations and policies for Internet gambling. The extent to which policies can be and are enforced also varies substantially between jurisdictions. Internet gambling regulation has not been in place for an extensive period of time making it difficult to isolate and measure its effectiveness. The lack of evidence on the impacts of various regulatory regimes increases the difficulties for policy makers, governments and regulators to enact the most appropriate strategies to regulate Internet gambling (Gainsbury and Wood 2011).

Although there are two main regulatory options, prohibition and legalisation, there are substantial variations in the ways in which governments can enact these policies.

Prohibition

Prohibition attempts to restrict residents from using Internet gambling and Internet gambling operators from supplying services to residents. Examples of jurisdictions that have adopted a policy of prohibition include the US, China, New Zealand, Japan and Thailand. Prohibition may be based on moral grounds, to protect land-based operators who have paid licence fees for the right to trade in specific geographic areas, or to limit the availability of gambling. Prohibition legislation can target Internet gamblers, online gambling providers, or financial institutions. Various measures are utilised by jurisdictions to enforce prohibitions on online gambling (Department of Broadband Communications and the Digital Economy, DBCDE 2011).

Blocking Financial Transactions

Several countries have introduced legislation to block financial transactions to online gambling providers. Such regulation requires banks and financial institutions to block payments based on Merchant Category Codes that are identified as gambling operators. In the US, banks and credit card companies are restricted from processing transactions for Internet gambling sites and it is illegal for Internet gambling operators to accept money from gamblers based in the US. In France, the gambling regulator can order the freezing of transactions relating to bank accounts identified as belonging to unlicensed operators. In Norway, payments from Norwegian cards to unlicensed online gambling operators are blocked and the Norwegian Gaming Authority may also order the refusal of transactions to and from particular bank accounts. This may be an effective deterrent as it would allow Dutch residents to claim back any losses, making it unprofitable for online gambling sites to provide services to these customers. However, in some cases, such measure may be expensive and resource intensive, with a number of methods available to bypass the controls reducing their effectiveness. Online gambling transactions are often difficult to identify and can be easily masked by gambling providers to avoid detection. Customers can also use third party payment methods to avoid recognition of sources of funds transfers.

Blocking Access to Online Gambling Websites

Governments can also attempt to block access to online gambling websites through regulation that forces Internet service providers to detect and block these sites. Such filters seek to ensure that potential customers are prevented from accessing unauthorised pre-listed sites. Internet Protocol (IP) blocking is another method in which the connection between a server or website and IP addresses within a specified domain (such as geographical domains) is blocked. These measures are used to support prohibition in China and Thailand and to support regulated access in France, Italy and Denmark (DBCDE 2011). Failure to block access to online gambling sites can result in fines and having operating licences revoked. However, individuals can use proxy servers to circumvent restrictions imposed by geolocation software and avoid having their location disclosed. The efficiency of blocking systems also is dependent on the comprehensive identification of all sites and servers to be blocked as well as efficient software systems that are regularly updated.

Criminal Sanctions and Fines

A number of jurisdictions *impose criminal sanctions and fines* for the provision of online gambling to residents. Recent actions have been taken by US authorities against online gambling operators (described below). In China online gambling operators have been successfully prosecuted, fined and received jail terms (Beach 2009). It is also illegal for citizens to gambling online and individuals can be penalised (DBCDE 2011). However, it can be difficult to prosecute offshore gambling operators who may be based in jurisdictions that will not cooperate with local authorities and law enforcement. Some sites are operated relatively anonymously making it difficult to identify and track the operators. For example, in the period from July 2010 to June 2011, the Australian Communication and Media Authority completed 48 investigations of allegations of operators providing Internet gambling illegally to Australian residents (DBCDE 2011). Yet, no operator has been prosecuted for violating Australia's Interactive Gambling Act, which has a limited range of enforcement options, despite penalties of AUD\$220,000 per day for individuals and AUD\$1.1 million per day for corporations.

Effectiveness of Prohibition

Evidence indicates that in many jurisdictions that have attempted to prohibit Internet gambling, many residents are still gambling online. For example, 91% of sites accept play from Australia, 89% accept play from China and 41% accept play from the US, despite policies prohibiting online gambling in these jurisdictions (Casino City Online 2011). In a study of 1,920 online gamblers who responded to advertisements on gambling sites, 87% originated from the US (Wood and Williams 2007), indicating that customers are interested and actively pursuing online gambling options. Similarly, in Norway, despite legislative efforts to block financial transactions to offshore gambling sites, it is estimated that 4% of Norweigians over the age of 18 gamble on foreign websites (Peppin 2011a). Ontario's Finance Minster Dwight Duncan claimed that over CAD\$400 million was being spent by Canadians on foreign sites in justification for the need for a province-based Internet gambling site (Parness 2010). Similarly, AUD\$968 million was estimated to be spent by Australians on offshore casino, bingo and poker sites in 2010 (Productivity Commission 2010).

Some of the difficulties in enforcing prohibition are outlined above. In general, it is difficult to limit the Internet sites that can be accessed by technologically savvy individuals, it is difficult to prosecute offshore operators located in foreign jurisdictions and effective measures are expensive and require constant monitoring and updating to keep pace with the Internet gambling industry. In 2011, the Australian Federal Policy acknowledged that since 2009, 15 allegations of criminal breaches of the Interactive Gambling Act, which prohibits online gambling, have not been investigated due to a lack of resources (Smith 2011). Most measures to enforce prohibition are relatively easy to circumvent by individuals intent on gambling online. A simple Google search results in many sites (e.g., wikiHow. com) that contain instructions for individuals that wish to circumvent bans on Internet gambling. A potential negative impact of prohibition is that by blocking reputable sites that are more likely to obey jurisdictional requirements, the market is left open for disreputable sites, located in jurisdictions with few restrictions or requirements, that arguable offer a greater risk to players (Eadington 2004; McMillen 2000; Rose 2008).

Legalisation and Licensing

Regulation may authorize governments to license gambling operators and enable them to provide residents of that jurisdiction access to online gambling sites. This may result in significant tax revenue from the gaming operator and at the same time aim to provide a fully regulated product to protect the consumer. Increased liberalisation of Internet gambling regulation has played a key role in the rapid growth of online gambling and this growth is expected to continue with increased levels of participation accompanying further legalisation. Levels of regulation can vary substantially between jurisdictions in terms of the codes of conduct required and extent to which operators are monitored and required to comply with specific regulations.

Closed Regulation

In closed regulatory systems, such as Italy, France, and the Netherlands, licenses and advertising rights are limited to domestic providers, which must be located within their country's geographical boundaries and these are only permitted to offer some types of products (Holliday 2011). Recent announcements suggest that Dutch legislation may be modified to grant licenses and allow foreign competition, again demonstrating the dynamic nature of Internet gambling policies (Reuters 2011).

Open Regulation

Open regulatory systems, such as that in the UK, allows Internet gambling service providers based in international jurisdictions to provide services to domestic residents. Further variations exist within these broad categories, for example, in Australia there is a combination of prohibition and open regulation; Internet gambling providers are not permitted to accept play from Australian residents, so must look offshore for customers, although online wagering and lotteries are permitted provided that they are licensed within Australia (Gainsbury 2010).

Government Ownership

Some jurisdictions, for example Norway, Sweden and Canada, legalise and regulate online gambling, but this is limited to a single site that is owned by the government. Under such an approach, the government becomes the operator and regulator and all revenues are returned to the government. Under these circumstances, there is an enhanced moral obligation to implement tighter, more restrictive policies and ensure that corporate social responsibility measures are in place. Within this framework, government is not only regulating and licensing its own online gambling but endorsing and providing tacit encouragement to its citizens to participate. The Canadian province of Ontario has also applied an effective framework in their implementation of an Internet gambling platform (to be launched in 2012) (Gainsbury and Blaszczynski 2011b). The site will not be launched until extensive consultation with stakeholders has been completed and a strict responsible gambling platform will be introduced based on empirical evidence and consultation with stakeholders. Among the responsible gambling tools to be included are mandatory limits for time and money, pop-up messages to communicate with players, self-help tests and information about games and self-exclusion options for various periods of time.

Offshore Licensing

Some jurisdictions, such as Alderney, Gibraltar, Norfolk Island and Kahnawake, license operators of online gambling sites with the primary intention of providing online gambling to offshore jurisdictions. The Alderney Gambling Control Commission (AGCC) provides an example of a successful regulatory framework for Internet gambling and has a highly regard reputation within the Internet casino industry. Operating since 2002, in 2010 Alderney generated a profit of AUD$5.8 million in licensing fees from Internet casinos, which, combined with other income generated from online gambling, was utilised to benefit local communities such as building an old age home (Cass 2011). The regulatory objectives of the AGCC are to:

- Ensure that funding, management and operations remains free from criminal influence;
- Ensure that eGambling is conducted honestly and fairly; and
- Protect the interests of public (children and vulnerable) (Wilsenach 2011).

The licensing and activation process is based on thorough testing of the suitability of the application including the applicant's character, business reputation, financial position, ownership and corporate structure, character and reputation of business associates and sources of funding. Furthermore, the business processes, equipment and product are tested and approved. Following licensing there is ongoing compliance checks with the regulatory requirements through monitoring and reviews, inspections, customer complaints, 'mystery shopping exercises' and special investigations where necessary. Disciplinary sanctions are enforced if sites and operators do not comply with regulations.

Impact of Legalisation on Participation Rates

By legalizing and regulating Internet gambling, governments are providing tacit approval for this activity, and citizens may make the assumption that it is a safe product (Gainsbury 2010). Increased availability of gambling opportunities typically results in a simultaneous increase in gambling behaviour and problem gambling (National Research Council 1999; Productivity Commission 2010). Constant availability of gambling from any location, accompanied by increased in advertising may normalise this activity, resulting in increased participation and less perception of potential harms (Monaghan and Derevensky 2008). This is particularly of concern for adolescents, who are highly influenced by advertising (Monaghan et al. 2009).

In most jurisdictions, liberalization of online gambling would not increase individual's ability to access both unsafe and safe international websites (Productivity Commission 2010). However, although prohibition does not appear to be effective in preventing all individuals from gambling online it is possible that legalizing and regulating Internet gambling would increase participation. Jurisdictions where Internet gambling is legalized and regulated have higher participation rates; for example, 6.5% of the adult population gambles online in Norway and 13% in the UK (Sandven 2007; Wardle et al. 2011b). In British Columbia, 20% of those with Internet access reported visit the provincially-operated PlayNow website once a month or more often (Tromp 2011). Nonetheless, surveys conducted in Australia and Nevada report that non-Internet gamblers are not gambling online due to the regulatory regimes, but for other reasons, and they would not be likely to start gambling online if policies were changed (Allen Consulting Group 2003; Bernhard et al. 2007). As the number of people with Internet access is expected to increase, it is likely that the number of online gambling sites and governments operating or regulating and licensing such sites will likely continue to escalate. Ultimately, this will result in a significant increase in the number of individuals gambling via the Internet.

Effectiveness of Regulation

It has been argued that it may not be possible to regulate Internet gambling to the same standards that can be set for land-based gambling (McMillen 2000; Wood and Williams 2007). There has yet to be a satisfactory model proposed, outlining how jurisdictional regulators would ensure that all sites meet minimum standards of satisfactory business and responsible gambling practices, and prevent citizens from using unregulated sites that do not offer appropriate player protection or abide by taxation laws (Gainsbury and Wood 2011). The administrative and enforcement costs of monitoring Internet gambling regulation and compliance are likely to be significant (Allen Consulting Group 2003).

The long-term effectiveness of regulated online gambling will depend on the ability of a jurisdiction to effectively deal with illegal competition (Gainsbury 2010). To date, the enforcement of bans on offshore or unlicensed operators has been very limited internationally, mainly due to the fact that remote operators offering illegal services to residents are located abroad. Jurisdictions that wish to enforce a closed regulatory system or protect a monopoly the measures that can be used are similar to those used to prohibit Internet gambling. In jurisdictions that permit foreign operators to obtain licences, there are some measures that can be enacted to encourage major international operators to comply with regulations. For example, the right to offer the product to residents and advertise in certain jurisdictions may be conditional on meeting standards for harm-minimization (as in the UK). Furthermore, public education campaigns can encourage consumers to play only on regulated sites and increase awareness of the potential risks associated with unregulated sites.

However, overly restrictive regulations may not be effective given the high level of competition from offshore sites and the relative ease of access that consumers have to these. For example, a study of the German market showed that the restrictive regulations in place (prohibition of private providers and advertising in favour of state-owned monopolies) have resulted in sharp revenue declines, the predominate use of online gambling offers from abroad, massive revenue losses for state-run gambling providers and high financial decline for the German state (Gold Media 2010). Similarly, restrictions, complicated technical requirements and high taxation in France appears to have benefited the illegal offshore market, which represents 57% of the entire online gambling market in France (European Gaming and Betting Association, EGBA 2011). In contrast, the Italian government has optimised the taxation system for online gambling and as a result has limited the illegal market, resulting in an increased state budget with total income from games doubled between 2003 and 2009 (EGBA 2011). These results indicate that a careful balance is required in regulation to legalise and license online gambling to enable legal sites to be competitive with offshore sites in order to capture an appropriate market share.

Taxation

There appear to be strong economic incentives that are encouraging governments to legalize and regulated Internet gambling, particularly during an economic downturn or recession. Gambling is a significant source of government revenue, which is often used for social benefits, including supporting cultural, sports, health and education. Gambling revenues have increased dramatically with an increase in legalized gaming opportunities, availability and accessibility. Just 15 years since the first online gambling site, the global Internet gambling industry is worth €24 billion (Holliday 2011). The online gambling sector appears to have benefitted from the global financial crisis of the late 2000s with positive growth is still occurring in this market (Mangion 2010).

Prohibition results in revenues moving offshore to foreign-owned sites, with taxes collected by foreign governments (Productivity Commission 2010). Legalised Internet gambling would establish an appropriate taxation model resulting in taxation revenue returning to the federal and state governments and the community through funding of research, prevention and treatment schemes from government and industry bodies (Gainsbury 2010). Funds can also be redirected to sporting and racing bodies that provide products on which bets are placed. A tax-revenue analysis conducted by Price Waterhouse Coopers concluded that taxation of Internet gambling in the US alone would be expected to generate between US$8.7–$42.8 billion in federal revenues over a 10 year period (Sandman 2008). More recently, Washington Democratic Representative Jim McDermott estimated that US$72 billion (US$42 billion federally and $30 billion for state governments) could be raised over 10 years through taxing online operators and gambling winnings (Benston 2010). Half of this amount would come from gamblers declaring taxable winnings, a model not used in many parts of the world, and it is questionable how compliance would be enforced. Furthermore, licensing Internet gambling encourages, and in some cases requires, operators to establish residence or at least corporate offices within the jurisdiction, which has the effect of keeping money within the country. A portion of taxation revenue should be directed towards treatment, prevention, and ongoing research to evaluate and monitor the impacts of Internet gambling and the effectiveness of responsible gambling policies and harm minimization tools (Gainsbury 2010).

Despite the potential economic benefits of legalized Internet gambling, governments may become dependent upon Internet gambling revenue, creating a conflict of interest that reduces their ability to deal with problem gambling (Anglican Diocese of Melbourne Social Responsibilities Committee 2008; Crumb 2010; Pulsipher 2005). This has already become evident for land-based casinos and gambling in some jurisdictions such as the gambling Meccas of Nevada, Atlantic City, and Biloxi, where gambling declines are resulting in serious economic problems for governments and their related spending (Crumb 2010). Conflicts of interest may be reduced by establishing an independent body to regulate Internet gambling and provide funding for research, prevention and treatment as in Canada.

Where markets are open, legalising Internet gambling will increase the competitiveness of sites. Given that competition is primarily realized through price competition (bonuses, payoff ratios, house cuts, etc.), it may become more difficult for some sites to survive as there are always other companies willing to reduce the price as long as the lower price still covers marginal costs (Eadington 2004). For these reasons, capturing "economic rents" through excise taxes on online gambling might be difficult for policymakers to achieve, particularly as it is presumed that regulated sites would have higher costs than unregulated sites with fewer consumer protection practices. There may also be a tendency for regional or national governments to "price compete" on tax rates against one another (Eadington 2004). This is evident from a report compiled by international experts advising South Africa on appropriate regulatory policy that suggested they offer more favourable tax rates than in Australia in order to capture a greater proportion of the market share (National Centre for Academic Research into Gaming 1999).

Within Europe, Germany's proposed 16.7% levy on the turnover of wagering operators was met with harsh criticism from the gambling industry (Goodley 2011). It was suggested that the high tax rate would mean that there would be little tax collected as companies would not be able to offer competitive products and would choose not to operate in the country. The online gambling market in France has encountered challenges in attracting operators due to the business environment and tax rates ('Online sports betting' 2011). It has been argued that Internet gambling sites would benefit from being licensed within a particular jurisdiction, as this would signal to potential customers that they adhere to the appropriate standards and are accountable to jurisdictional laws, and hence the sites would be prepared to pay taxes. In a ruling in relation to Denmark, the European Commission confirmed that member states are entitled under EU state aid rules to apply lower tax rates to online compared to land-based gambling activities ('State aid' 2011). The rationale stated for the ruling was that the positive effects of the liberalisation of the online gambling sector outweighed potential distortions of competition and taxes "making the Danish online providers too expensive would have rendered the liberalisation of the market devoid of purpose" ('State aid' 2011). This ruling recognises the importance of a business model that enables online operators to compete in this market and that excessively high duties would not increase revenue as players are likely to turn to illegal sites.

Regulators and Internet gambling operators internationally have faced conflicts over the most appropriate taxation rates. McDermott's proposed bill in the US included a deposit tax where money deposited into gambling accounts would be taxed regardless of whether it was gambled, which is argued to collect taxes from companies without having to work out where customers are based and reduce the differences between online operators and land-based venues, which have greater overhead costs (Benston 2010). Betting companies prefer to be taxed on their gross profits – that is, the profits that they make from gamblers, rather than turnover (Goodley 2011). Turnover is classified as the total amount of money staked with a bookmaker, but that figure includes money that a successful gambler has won. For example, a winning $5 bet at 2-1 would earn a gambler $15; if he then bets the $15 and loses, he makes a net loss of $5. Under a gross profits tax the bookmaker would be taxed on the $5. Under a turnover tax, it is taxed on both bets, that is, $20. Following a comprehensive review of gambling, the Australian Productivity Commission (2010) concluded that gross revenue/profits appears to be the more appropriate basis upon which product fees should be charged. This method is already widely used internationally and can be applied universally without disproportionately burdening certain types of operators and is likely to deliver better value to consumers and a wider range of products. In some jurisdictions various online operators pay different taxes and fees. For example, in Australia, corporate bookmakers may pay different tax rates to totalisators and betting exchanges. However, a Federal Court decision in June 2011, ruled in favour of Sportsbet, suggesting that the NSW racing bodies had imposed turnover fees (1.5% on gambling turnover) that were discriminating in favour of the monopoly totalisator, Tabcorp (Bennett 2011a). This was ruled protectionist, discriminatory and unlawful and Racing NSW was ordered to repay Sportsbet AU$2 million. A similar case involving Betfair Australia and relating to the right to use race fields information has now been taken to the Australian High Court. These examples demonstrate the importance of considering the relevant contributions of all operators and the benefits allocated to each (e.g., physical retail outlets, advertising rights, rights to offer bets on various events) to ensure, as much as possible, a level playing field.

Revenue may still move offshore if foreign-owned or offshore regulated sites are allowed to operate within a jurisdiction. For example, the UK has a White List of sites that are permitted to offer online gambling, even if these are regulated offshore, such as in Alderney or the Isle of Man, which favours offshore operators as these pay lower taxes (Church-Sanders 2011). Gamblers are sometimes required to report gambling winnings and pay tax on these revenues, for example in the US (Hammer 2001). Individuals winning money by gambling online may avoid reporting taxable winnings due to cross-jurisdictional regulations. It is uncertain whether they should pay tax on money won from the jurisdiction where the site is located or one's residence. In summary, the taxation model implemented in relation to Internet gambling must be carefully considered by regulators to ensure that onshore gambling sites can be competitive with the offshore market and still contribute appropriate levels of funds to governments, the community, and appropriate sport and racing bodies.

Impact on Existing Industries

Liberalisation of Internet gambling may threatened existing gambling operators as well as related businesses including the travel, hospitality and entertainment industries (Hammer 2001). This may result in associated reduction in tax revenue from existing industries, including land-based gambling. It has been argued that increased use of Internet gambling will draw money from other businesses as opposed to stimulating the economy (Eadington 1995; Grinols 2001), although these arguments assume a finite amount of money. The Australian Productivity Commission (2010) noted that to remain competitive with other international jurisdictions, online gambling sites would have to be taxed at lower rates than terrestrial operators. In addition to not having to pay overheads associated with having a physical venue, this would allow online operators to provide gambling opportunities with lower costs to consumers as compared to land-based venues, which may have an impact on existing operators, particularly those that do not provide online betting options.

However, European reports indicate that the growth of Internet gambling is not detrimental to the traditional offline segment, which is expected to retain the vast majority of the total gambling market and continue to grow in revenue (EGBA 2011). For example, in Italy, lottery turnover has continued to grow (from €15.8 billion in 2007 to €19.5 billion in 2010) concurrently with the growth in the online sports betting and poker market (€1.1 billion in 2007 to €4.8 billion in 2010; EGBA 2011). Similarly, in the UK, which is one of the most competitive and open online gambling markets in the world, the National Lottery announced record ticket sales of £5.8bn in the year to March 2011, representing an increase of 6.8% on the previous year (Camelot 2011). However, it should be noted that lottery ticket sales are available online and interactive sales grew during this period, demonstrating that traditional land-based gambling operators can take advantage of the trend in online gambling.

The small amount of available research indicates that the majority of Internet gamblers are active in multiple forms of gambling (AGA 2006; Griffiths et al. 2009a; Wood and Williams 2010), indicating that increased participation in online gambling may not lead to a concomitant reduction of land-based gambling activities. Australian research reported that approximately 50% of Internet gambling turnover is replacing gambling through more traditional means, such as telephone betting, and around 50% represents additional gambling activity (Allen Consulting Group 2003). However, in this context this substitution may represent different modes of betting with the same operator. Further, this survey found that all respondents who were Internet gamblers had previously engaged in a more traditional form of gambling. The majority (76%) of Australian Internet gamblers surveyed in 2003 believed that their Internet gambling was likely to remain stable over the next few years (Allen Consulting Group 2003). However, 16% reported that their thought their Internet gambling would increase, compared to 7% who thought that it would decrease over time. A survey of Internet gamblers in the US indicated that Internet gamblers may increase their level of gambling 50% upon legalisation, and even increase play at land-based venues by a small amount (AGA 2006). Among Nevada residents, four out of five online gamblers surveyed reported that gambling online had not affected their gambling in conventional settings (Bernhard et al. 2007). A more recent survey in Canada found that 68% of respondents indicated that Internet gambling does not affect how often they visit a casino and the remaining 32% were evening divided on whether Internet gambling would increase or decrease their casino visitation (Ipsos Reid 2010). However, it is likely those who gamble online currently, including on unregulated sites, are more driven and interested in online gambling than the general public and their behaviour does not accurately predict how the wider public would act if Internet gambling is legalised.

The gaming industry is a major employer that could potentially be hurt by reduced land-based gambling, although, it has been argued that there are additional jobs associated with Internet gambling. For example, Washington Democrat Congress representative, Jim McDermott, estimated legalization of Internet gambling in the US would create 32,000 jobs (Benston 2010). Similarly, a Swedish study indicated that liberalisation of the online gambling market and regulation would lead to considerable job creation (EGBA 2011). Furthermore, the jobs created require highly skilled individuals', which is expected to promote higher training and ongoing education in addition to ongoing research to continually advance digital technologies, making an important contribution to jurisdictions' innovation and e-commerce in general. The Internet gambling industry has links to other sectors of the economy, such as information technology and communications, which may benefit from increased Internet gambling due to increased demand (Allen Consulting Group 2003).

The racing industry is particularly vulnerable to any substitution towards overseas Internet gambling, or online operators that do not contribute to the racing industry (Allen Consulting Group 2003). Concerns have been raised over potential "free-riding" whereby online gambling operators allow betting on markets to which they do not financially contribute (European Commission 2011a; Productivity

Commission 2010). However, in regulated markets, Internet gambling operators appear to be supportive of policies that mandate a certain proportion of profits are returned to support sports and racing industries, provided that this proportion is fair and reasonable for all regulated operators (EGBA 2011; Productivity Commission 2010). Online gambling appears to be creating additional sources of revenue for sports and racing in terms of corporate sponsorship and advertising, including community, grass-roots level and amateur sports. For example, gambling-related funds have made a substantial contribution to revenue-raising for host cities of Olympic Games, including Italy and London (EGBA 2011).

Overall, the conclusion is mixed on the economic impact of liberalised Internet gambling regulation. Factors to consider include:

- The extent to which Internet gambling industry will benefit in terms of increased revenue;
- Whether the competitive pressures created by online providers will increase cost effectiveness of land-based gambling and whether existing forms of gambling will suffer;
- Overseas providers will compete (legally or illegally) for market share with local providers and may be able to offer better odds as they can avoid tax obligations;
- The impact on the sports and racing industry and appropriate product fees and taxes to balance economic impacts to sustain these industries;
- Benefits to businesses associated with Internet gambling, including increased technological capacity, skills and research to advance the jurisdiction;
- Whether other industries may suffer with expenditure re-directed to Internet gambling.

Payment Processors and Credit Cards are Impacted by Online Gambling Regulation

There are currently around 200 payment methods used by Internet gambling sites worldwide (Casino City Online 2011), and credit cards, eWallets and money transfers appear to be the most popular (Church-Sanders 2011; Wood and Williams 2010). A safe and secure payment system for online gambling, through a native financial institution, is considered to be a key factor in regional online gambling market growth (KPMG 2010). The UIGEA laws in the US require financial institutions and payment processors to identify and block monetary transfers to online gambling sites from US citizens (Church-Sanders 2011). The US Treasury estimated that it would take payment providers one million hours to implement the policies and procedures required to bring them into compliance with the rules, at a cost of over US$100 million in the first year (Church-Sanders 2011).

Internet gambling places banks and credit card companies in a precarious position (Hammer 2001). These institutions can profit greatly by offering credit to individuals to gamble online. Credit card charges for Internet gambling are often posted as cash advances, which carry higher interest rates than ordinary purchases. However, numerous lawsuits and bankruptcy declarations have been filed by individuals who have lost money gambling and who refuse to pay gambling debts (Hammer 2001). These lawsuits could leave banks unable to collect debts from individuals who partake in Internet gambling or force individuals into bankruptcy. If Internet gamblers are successful in having their debts alleviated, non-Internet gamblers will ultimately pay the costs in terms of higher fees, charges and interest rates passed onto all credit card holders (Hammer 2001). Most credit cards charge higher rates of interest for cash purchases and a UK study suggests that all of the large credit card firms in the UK are treating online gambling deposits as cash advances, with interest rates as high as 27.95%, a fact understood by few gamblers ('Credit cards' 2011). Banks are increasingly aware of online gambling and are tracking these transactions. For example, although online gambling is not prohibited in Ireland, payments to online betting operators are being used as reasons for refusing bank loans and mortgages as this is viewed as a non-essential activity (Hennessry 2011).

Credit and electronic payment methods are also causing some difficulties for online gambling operators. Leading international gambling consultants have identified credit cards as a key area of concern for the industry (KPMG 2010). By making it easier for players to deposit money and not completing customer due diligence, operators can increase their bad debt levels. For example, PartyGaming reported that the amount of customer bad debts rose 190% between 2008 and 2009, from US$2.1 million to US$6.1 million, representing 1.4% of PartyGaming's total 2009 revenues (Bad debts rise 2011). The charge-off rate on bad debts by credit card firms rose significantly in 2009, causing firms to raise fees and interest rates in response to bad debts during the recent recession (KPMG 2010). This could cause considerable difficulties for online gambling companies, who rely on customers being able to transfer funds to use their products. Several online gambling operators have reported increased payment processing costs and bad debts since 2009 (Bad debts rise 2011). For example, 888 Holdings reported that its chargeback expenses rose 87.5% from US$4.82 million to US$9.04 million between 2008 and 2009, representing 4.6% of net gaming revenues ('Bad debts rise' 2011). Issues relating to electronic payment methods are likely to continue as new payment processing options are developed, particularly in relation to mobile gambling and operators enter markets without well developed Internet banking systems.

Social Costs

Although governments can take action to mitigate and minimize the social costs associated with Internet gambling, it is important to note that this form of gambling is not without risks (Gainsbury 2010). Current estimates suggest that between 1% and 5% of adults in the general population meet criteria for problem or pathological gambling (Abbott 2007; Petry 2005; Productivity Commission 2010; Reith 2006;

Wardle et al. 2011b). Some evidence suggests that these rates are decreasing in response to consumer protection policies, responsible gambling strategies, and/or social adaptation (LaPlante and Shaffer 2007; Shaffer and Martin 2011). However, the trend toward legalization of Internet gambling and concomitant increased availability, promotion and widespread market penetration are anticipated to lead to a resurgent incidence of problem gambling (Abbott et al. 2004; Grun and McKeigue 2000; National Research Council 1999; Toneatto and Ladouceur 2003; Welte et al. 2009). In addition to the significant negative impacts experienced by individuals, their friends and families, problem gambling has a large social cost related to lost productivity and work disruption, unemployment, family breakdown, mental and physiological health problems, legal and financial difficulties, crime, bankruptcy, and suicide. For example, the annual social cost of problem gambling in Australia is estimated at AUD$4.7 billion, excluding some immeasurable costs such as those relating to suicide (Productivity Commission 2010).

Internet gambling has been repeatedly linked with higher rates of problem gambling (Focal Research Consultants 2008; South Australian Centre for Economic Studies 2008; Volberg et al. 2006; Wood and Williams 2007, 2010; Wood et al. 2007). A causal connection has not been established and it is likely that Internet gambling acts to create new problems for some individuals, and to exacerbate and maintain existing problems for others (Wood and Williams 2010). It is critical than any regulatory policies take account the likelihood of increases in associated gambling problems in the community. If governments make efforts to legalize and regulate Internet gambling, it is important that they do so only with a realistic appreciation of the concomitant social costs (Gainsbury 2010; Gainsbury and Wood 2011; Wood and Williams 2007). Appropriate longitudinal research is needed to determine the social impact of legalised Internet gambling.

In addition to the potential increase in the incidence of problem gambling, governments and regulators should consider the response from citizens. In some countries, for example, Canada and Australia, governments have faced significant criticisms and accusations of relying on gambling revenues at the cost of individual problem gamblers (Gainsbury and Wood 2011). Some jurisdictions face substantial opposition to the expansion of gambling based on moral beliefs or a sense that people are being harmed by excessive gambling. For example, key findings from American gambling attitude surveys indicate that far more Americans believe that gambling's effect on society are negative rather than positive and public concerns increase in relation to gambling expansion (Pew Research Center 2006; Toce-Gerstein and Gerstein 2007). Negative attitudes towards gambling and concerns about the expansion of gambling and gambling-related harm also appear prevalence in jurisdictions with heavy gambling availability, including Australia, the UK, and Macau (Smith et al. 2011). In a sample of 1,808 Canadians from one province, Smith et al. (2011) found that casino gambling via the Internet was viewed as the most harmful form of gambling and bingo and sports pools on the Internet were ranked as the 7th and 8th most harmful forms out of 16. Similarly, a Newspoll survey conducted in Australia reported that 63% of respondents believed advertising by sports betting agencies (one of the only forms of legal online gambling in

Australia) increased problem gambling and 42% believed that giving the gambling odds during live sports coverage should be illegal (Australian Associated Press 2011). Therefore, any changes in regulation to increase access to Internet gambling may result in more negative attitudes from citizens.

Politicians and regulators can take steps to reduce the potential negative impacts of Internet gambling by building specific measures into any legalisation policies. Online gambling operators must have a high standard of consumer protection measures in place and responsible gambling strategies, such as those discussed in a later chapter. At a community level, public education advertisements should inform the population about the risks of online gambling, particularly those associated with unregulated sites. Funds should be collected directly from online operators, in addition to funds from taxes that must contribute to ongoing research to measure the impact of online gambling at a societal level and the most effective responsible gambling measures to be implemented. In addition, policy makers must allocate specific funds for treatment and prevention programs specifically for Internet gambling.

Inter-Jurisdictional Considerations

The technological transformation calls into question traditional models of gambling regulation that concentrate on controlling market entry (through licensing and regulation) and gambling transactions (through surveillance and auditing) (McMillen 2000). The nature of online gambling means that it operates outside the traditional restraints of jurisdictional borders, which presents both challenges and opportunities for regulators (Gainsbury and Wood 2011). Although jurisdictions require different regulatory structures to suit their environment, international cooperation may be prudent to increase the effectiveness of individual policies, enable mutual protection of interests and reduce the burden on gambling operators licensed in multiple jurisdictions.

Some jurisdictions that regulate access to Internet gambling are exploring the possibility of entering into agreements, particularly those closely geographically located. In Canada, although each province regulates gambling independently, the provinces offering Internet gambling share a platform and enforce regional compliance by refusing play to residents of provinces that do not permit online gambling (Gainsbury and Wood 2011). This arrangement demonstrates the feasibility of collaborative arrangements, including revenue sharing and has benefits for customers by increasing the number of players against whom they can compete. The respective regulators of France and Italy have signed a memorandum of understanding to formalise information sharing and discuss common issues (DBCDE 2011). The regulators will seek to work together on regulatory issues, the control of legal operators and illegal sites, as well as fraud and consumer safety.

The benefits of aligning regulation with that of similar jurisdictions include the promotion of international consumer protection standards (Gainsbury 2010).

Given the multitude of different policies, it is very difficult for Internet gambling operators to abide by these for each jurisdiction; however, the use of a common set of guidelines would make it easier for operators to comply and jurisdictions to enforce regulation. In particular it is important that a common set of regulations be used across a country wherever possible to avoid inter-jurisdictional disputes. For example, in Canada and Australia individual state policies differ, causing competition between these jurisdictions and difficulties in terms of advertising, products permitted and taxation. A national regulatory body would more easily be able to regulate and monitor online gambling sites and for operators to ensure that they abide by rules (Productivity Commission 2010). It would avoid the duplication of resources and services and allow a central consumer protection body to operate and investigate any complaints or regulatory breaches (Gainsbury 2010). Cooperative policy options include mutual recognition or harmonization. Under mutual recognition, a gaming operator complying with the requirements of his jurisdiction of origin has the right to provide his services in all other jurisdictions under the regulatory framework. Under harmonization, all different jurisdictional rules would be replaced by a single set of harmonised rules. Compliance with the harmonised licensing requirements would then be sufficient to gain access in another member jurisdiction (Vlaemminck and De Wael 2003).

The European Commission's 2011 Green Paper on on-line gambling recommended that possible areas of administrative co-operation include sharing or exchanging information relating to:

- License holders, including licence conditions, professional qualities of staff and integrity of operators;
- Unlicensed and fraudulent operators, that is, common blacklisting;
- Technical issues, such as national standards, testing and certification;
- Best practices, including public campaigns to prevent crime or problem gambling and the costs and effects of such campaigns.

Gambling authorities may also benefit from working cooperatively to develop educational programs or campaigns for athletes, coaches, referees, and all persons employed in professions that give them inside information and/or an opportunity to influence the outcome of games. In addition, the joint development of early warning systems and identification of suspicious betting patterns may strengthen the enforcement of match-fixing.

The CEN Workshop (2010), incorporating members of the national standards bodies of 30 European and Mediterranean countries, developed nine draft control objectives relating to responsible Internet gambling. The intent was to establish uniform guidelines, principles and policies. The nine control objectives include:

- The protection of vulnerable customers
- The prevention of underage gambling
- Zero tolerance of fraudulent and criminal behaviour
- Protection of customer privacy and safeguarding of information
- Prompt and accurate customer payments

- Fair gaming
- Ethical and responsible marketing
- Commitment to customer satisfaction and support
- Secure, safe and reliable operating environment

These objectives represent likely common goals that can be shared by online gambling operators. Differences may exist in the measures used by online gambling operators to achieve the desired levels of consumer protection. The goal of harmonisation would be to negotiate between regulators and operators to achieve the appropriate level of protection.

Jurisdictional Base for Internet Gambling Sites

Despite the regulatory stance taken by various jurisdictions, due to the global and remote nature of online gambling, operators can choose where they wish their sites to be based and licensed, which may be offshore from their primary market. An offshore operator is defined as an operator that has its servers in a country where online gambling is licensed, but where players tend not to be based (Church-Sanders 2011). Factors considered by gambling operators include:

- Availability of licenses for various forms of Internet gambling;
- The regulatory structure, which may be reputable and set high standards of integrity, thus increasing the legitimacy of a site, or have a low license cost, including the costs of satisfying license terms, which are not onerous in many cases. The ease of communication and competence of a regulatory body may also play a role in choosing a regulatory base;
- The stability of a political environment including tax rates;
- Reliable and inexpensive telecommunication facilities, adequate bandwidth and availability of leased lines and satellite communications and appropriate and qualified employees to manage operations;
- Ability to target key markets including any restrictions on advertising (Church-Sanders 2011; Ranade et al. 2006).

The majority of Internet gambling sites are registered in just a few jurisdictions. In August, 2011, there were 74 jurisdictions around the world that currently regulate Internet gambling (Casino City Online 2011). The jurisdictions with the greatest number of sites are:

1. Malta – 547 sites
2. Netherlands Antilles – 376 sites
3. Gibraltar – 304 sites
4. Costa Rica – 219 sites
5. Kahnawake – 173 sites
6. United Kingdom – 199 sites
7. Alderney – 112 sites

8. Italy – 69 sites
9. Antigua and Barbuda – 67 sites
10. Cyprus – 63 sites

Many of these jurisdictions have legalised online gambling as an economic development strategy for attracting investment and jobs in a non-polluting, technology-oriented industry (Stewart et al. 2006). For example, in the UK White Listed Isle of Man, the Internet gambling industry grew by 24% in 2010, providing a growing job market for skilled employees, making it one of the jurisdictions most successful industries ('Survey' 2011). Online gambling companies and employees are contributing to the economy in multiple ways, the island's business environment and technological capabilities are improving and taxes collected are also increasing, confirming the importance of the industry for the island.

Having an Internet gambling license does not necessarily imply compliance with certain quality standards or high levels of consumer protection. There is a general lack of transparency about the quality of and requirements for licenses across jurisdictions, creating difficulties for regulators and consumers as well as online gambling operators. The UK has made attempts to reduce confusion by creating a 'white list' of licensing jurisdictions that meet strict and transparent criteria. The extent to which consumers know where sites they play on are licensed and appreciate that playing on offshore sites generally leaves them with little legal protection and means of redress in case they are cheated or have any dispute is unknown.

Specific Jurisdictional Policies

Internet gambling regulation and policy is difficult to describe due to constant changes. The following presents a brief summary of the regulatory stances of several jurisdictions and the impacts as of August 2011 on Internet gambling. Jurisdictions that have adopted a variety of regulatory responses were chosen to highlight the outcome of several policy options. Table 3.1 provides a summary of Internet gambling policies in various international jurisdictions.

North America

United States

The Unlawful Internet Gambling Enforcement Act (UIGEA) of 2006 was passed in 2006 attached to a port security measure without discussion in the Senate. Prior to the act being passed there was little public support for prohibition of Internet gambling with polls indicating that between 70% and 85% of respondents opposed prohibition efforts (Catania 2011). The UIGEA restricts US payment processors

Table 3.1 Regulatory stance across international jurisdictions

Country	Internet gambling policy	Details
Pacific		
Australia	Licensed lottery and wagering permitted	Licensed lottery and wagering permitted
New Zealand	Prohibition	Online lottery ticket sales permitted
North America		
US	Prohibition	Internet gambling approved in Washington, D.C.
Canada	Monopoly	Provincially owned and operated gambling sites in some provinces
Mexico	Open market	No specific online gambling regulation
Europe		
Norway	Monopoly	
Sweden	Monopoly	
Finland	Monopoly	
Austria	Monopoly	
Germany	Monopoly	
Hungary	Monopoly	
France	Closed market	
Italy	Closed market	
Netherlands	Closed market	
Czech Republic	Closed market	
Estonia	Closed market	
Belgium	Closed market	
Croatia	Licensed wagering permitted	Sports betting only
Denmark	Open market proposed	
Greece	Regulated market for poker and casino sites	Sports betting still monopoly
UK	Open market	
Spain	Online gambling to be regulated	
Ireland	Licensed lottery and wagering permitted	No specific online gambling regulation
Estonia	Open market	
Poland	Prohibition	Sports betting permitted
Russia	Prohibition	
Asia		
Japan	Prohibition/Monopoly	Online race wagering permitted by single operator
Thailand	Prohibition	
China	Prohibition	
Philippines	Monopoly	
India	Closed market/prohibition	Online lottery and licenses in Sikkim
South Korea	Prohibition	
Africa		
South Africa	Prohibition	
Tanzania	Open market	Limited Tanzanian-language sites
Egypt	Open market	No specific online gambling regulation

(continued)

Table 3.1 (continued)

Country	Internet gambling policy	Details
Central and South America		
Panama	Closed market	
Argentina	Closed market	Prohibited in Buenos Aires, licencees only allowed to accept local players
Costa Rica	Open market	
Chile	Open market	
Brazil	Prohibition	

including banks, credit card companies and all money transmitting businesses from processing transactions for any Internet gambling sites (Kelly 2008). It is also illegal for Internet gambling providers to accept money transfers from US online gamblers. There are exemptions to the UIGEA, including between-state horse race betting, and other types of within-state online gambling such as lotteries, as long as it is not prohibited at the state level. It is also unclear whether this legislation applied to 'skill games', which some have argued includes poker. The exceptions to the UIGEA were viewed by the World Trade Organisation (WTO) as unfair trade protection practices resulting in the WTO imposing a US\$21 million annual trade sanction in favour for Antigua and Barbuda in November 2006, although the WTO has little power to enforce sanctions (Capone 2009). The WTO ruling implied that the US is acting in a discriminatory, improper and protectionist manner by disallowing international online gambling while it allows online gambling in the form of horse racing and other forms of gambling in the US (Catania, 201). The EU has also investigated filing a complaint with the WTO over the US's enforcement of the UIGEA (Capone 2009).

Before UIGEA, North American accounted for 50% of the Internet gambling market, however, in 2010, North America represented only 24% of the global online gambling market (Holliday 2010). In response to the UIGEA, Internet gambling operators either withdrew from the lucrative US market, for example publicly traded 888 and PartyGaming, or aggressively targeted this market to capture US players, such as PokerStars and Full Tilt Poker, which increased player volumes from 30% to nearly 60% (Church-Sanders 2011; Holliday 2010). Poker sites accepting play from the US reported an 82% increase in player volume in 2010, compared to non-US sites, which had little to no player growth (Holliday 2010). Although some online gambling sites do not accept players based in the US, international regulators in many jurisdictions, including the UK, Isle of Man, and Kahnawake, do not require operators to refrain from taking bets from US customers (Catania 2011). This may indicate that these jurisdictions to not agree with the US regarding the legality of Internet gambling and the scope of US law. Furthermore, not accepting US players would significantly reduce taxes, fees, jobs and other economic benefits.

On April 15, 2011, dubbed 'Black Friday', a federal criminal case was brought against the founders of the three largest online poker companies, PokerStars, Full Tilt Poker and Cereus (Absolute Poker/Ultimatebet) and a handful of others.

Allegations were made that the defendants had violated the UIGEA and engaged in bank fraud and money laundering in order to process transfers to and from their customers (McLaughlin and Jinks 2011). The US Department of Justice seized the .com internet addresses of the sites, froze bank accounts and are seeking jail terms for some of the site founders and executives and payment processors. Subsequently, there have been several arrests, some of the sites have been unfrozen and begun processing cash-outs, an estimated US$200 million in advertising and marketing in the US has been withdrawn. Full Tilt Poker's gambling license has been revoked by Alderney, and Cereus has declared bankruptcy (Brunker 2011; Chaivarlis 2011; Rovell 2011; 'The Impact of the FullTilt.com' 2011). US players have yet to had their deposits returned from Full Tilt, Absolute Poker or Ultimatebet and the jurisdictions that licensed these sites have not taken any specific actions on behalf of their players (Catania 2011).

Sites that have continued to accept play from the US have benefited from the indictments, although operating from alternate domains, and some of the sites have managed to recapture some of their high value players ('The Impact of the FullTilt. com' 2011). However, a substantial proportion of players appear to have withdrawn from the market due to a lack of confidence in playing online poker in the current climate ('The Impact of the FullTilt.com' 2011). In August 2011, the US Immigration and Customs Enforcement and Homeland Security Investigations seized an online bingo site, resulting in similar sites withdrawing from this market (Williams 2011). This further action against online gambling sites indicates that the US Government will continue to pursue US facing gambling operators that ignore US legislation.

The past few years have seen a range of efforts to legalise Internet gambling in the US from industry organisations, lobby groups and politicians. The Nevada Gaming Commission has approved an amendment to the state's gaming regulations that will enable guests to use mobile devices to gamble in their hotel rooms in addition to public areas ('Nevada approves in-room gambling' 2011). Several casinos, including the Venetian, M Resort, Hard Rock, and Tropicana provide customers with wireless devices for mobile wagering. Several regulatory bills have been introduced, for example, then-Senate Majority Leader Harry Reid (Nevada) attempted to pass an online poker bill through Congress in 2010, but the lack of industry unification and political support is still limiting the impact of such endeavours (Gros 2011a). Online poker has been legalised in Washington, D.C., where community consultations are currently occurring, Internet gambling bills have been passed in Nevada and Iowa, although neither specifically permits online gamblers to operate, and bills have been considered in Massachusetts, New Jersey and California. Three regulatory bills were introduced in 2011 including a bill by Representative Barney Frank (Massachusetts) with support from Representative Joe Barton (Texas) that would legalise a wide variety of online gambling activities (Gros 2011a). However, lobbyists indicated that these bills have not greatly increased the perceived importance of Internet gambling regulation in Congress, nor do they have much support from influential members of the gaming industry or trade associations (Krafcik 2011).

Public support for legalisation appears to be weak; a poll conducted in 2010 by Fairleigh Dickinson Public Mind found that two-thirds of Americans "oppose changing the law to permit people to place bets over the Internet" (Post 2010). In the first quarter of 2011, 52 different special interest groups spend an estimated US$3.93 million lobbying Internet gambling in Washington, D.C., down 12.4% compared to the preceding quarter (Krafcik 2011). The current Republican dominated Congress, known for its hostility toward Internet gambling regulation, have somewhat diminished lobbying efforts. Opponents of Internet gambling, including card rooms and Indian gaming operators based in California, the single largest Internet gambling market in the US, increased lobbying expenditure by 27.5% in the first quarter relative to the fourth (Krafcik 2011). Federal enforcement action targeting executives at PokerStars and Full Tilt Poker in April, 2011, resulted in further decreases in lobbying expenditure. Both businesses were heavy financial backers of the Interactive Gaming Council, a trade group that advocates for Internet gambling regulation and contributes to the Poker Player Alliance. Opponents and special interest groups with undeclared or neutral stances on the issue also decreased lobbying expenditures. Given the significant size of the potential market it is likely that further developments will continue.

Canada

Canadians are estimated to spend between US$700 million and US$1 billion annually on interactive gaming (Kelly 2008). Canadian federal law has been interpreted by provincial governments as allowing them to legally operate an Internet gambling website as long as the patronage is restricted to residents within their respective province (Gainsbury and Wood 2011). Subsequently, there have been several Canadian provincial forays into online gambling, lead by the Atlantic Lottery Corporation (ALC), which first offered Internet gambling in 2004 (BC Partnership for Responsible Gambling 2011). Currently, online gambling is also available in British Columbia and Quebec with a large degree of cooperation between the provincial gaming corporations (Wood 2010). A range of Internet gambling opportunities are available including sports betting, casino games, bingo, keno, themed interactive games such as hangman and mini-golf, lottery ticket sales, and several versions of poker. In August, 2010, the Ontario Lottery and Gaming Corporation (OLG) announced that it plans to launch an online gambling site in 2012, following an 18 month period of consultation and study (Canadian Press 2011). The remaining provinces have stated that they are exploring the possibilities of Internet gambling, however, statements from political leaders in Nova Scotia, Newfoundland and Labrador and Alberta indicated that these provinces will not be offering Internet gambling to residents in the immediate future (Gainsbury and Wood 2011).

The prevalence rate of Internet gambling in Canada remains relative low, estimated to be between 2% and 8% (Ipsos Reid 2010; Wood and Williams 2010). However, it seems that government expansion into Internet gambling may have had some impact. In British Columbia, the prevalence rate of Internet gambling is 5.0%, and ranges from 3.1% to 8.2% in the various Atlantic Provinces (Wood and Williams 2010). In a public opinion survey of 1,724 Canadians, only 39% of the general population stated that they thought Internet gambling was an acceptable form of entertainment, although 60% reported that it should be permitted with Government regulation (Ipsos Reid 2010). In addition to regulated Internet gambling, Canadians also use offshore sites, and were recently affected by the US's prosecutorial actions against several large online poker sites. In September 2011, a Canadian class-action lawsuit was launched against Full Tilt Poker in an effort to recover between CAD$5 million and CAD$10 million withheld from Canadian patrons since June (Moore 2011).

Certain Aboriginal groups have enacted their own gambling legislation. For example, the Kahnawake Gaming Commission (KGC) regulates 172 Internet gambling sites, making it one of the largest online gambling jurisdictions in the world (Online Casino City 2011). The Attorney General of Canada and Minister of Justice in Quebec has stated that the Kahnawake operations are illegal; however, this has not been tested in court (Lipton and Weber 2005). It has been reported that Canada's Ministry of Justice has considered various measures to stop online gaming sites operated by the KGC; however, no actions have been taken and their operation remains ongoing and highly profitable (Lipton and Weber 2005). Any attempt to shut down Kahnawake's licensees will result in a long judicial process likely to be determined by the Supreme Court of Canada.

Europe

The European Union's online gambling and betting market represented 45% of the world market share in 2010 (EGBA 2011). The EU online gambling market represents 11% of the total European gambling market and is expected to expand to account for 13% of the total market by 2012, making online gambling one of the fastest growing industries in Europe (EGBA 2011). The European Commission has considered several policy options, including whether it would pass regulation covering all types of gambling services, deal with some issues, while leaving others to national law, or not act at all (Vlaemminck and De Wael 2003). Currently, Internet gambling policy in the EU is largely left to individual Member States who are responsible for establishing and administering rules for their respective markets, based upon national needs and cultural preferences, including gambling services.

One of the biggest challenges in Europe is the allowance of cross-border online gambling and currently, many countries have focussed gambling reform activities within their own borders (KPMG 2010). As a result, Internet gambling markets, types of games offered, laws, regulations, restrictions and controls are very heterogeneous across Europe (Church-Sanders 2011). Europe includes both liberalised gambling markets, closed markets that permit Internet gambling sites restricted to play within their borders, monopolies with strict controls, as well as several offshore gambling jurisdictions that are popular with operators such as Gilbraltar, Malta, and Alderney (Church-Sanders 2011).

Under EU law, the basic principle is the free movement of services. European Court of Justice rulings have protected EU Member states from being forced to allow Internet gambling within their jurisdictions, although cautioned that policies must be well defined and consistent to avoid discriminatory restrictions (Church-Sanders 2011). Accordingly, regulations appear to be moving towards requiring online gambling operators to obtain multiple licences to operate across European jurisdictions, representing a significant cost and effort for operators (Church-Sanders 2011). The EU Financial Services department is conducting a review of gaming laws across the region and in 2011 released a Green Paper on Online Gambling (White 2011).

The EU has recently expressed doubts regarding the compatibility of several draft Member States gambling laws with EU legal principles, rejecting their potentially discriminatory character (World Online Gambling Law Report 2011). Several governments in Europe have been resistant to liberalised gambling legislation, instead favouring restrictive measures and existing monopolies (Church-Sanders 2011). The European Commission has subsequently been investigating Greece, Norway, Germany, Sweden, the Netherlands, and France (Church-Sanders 2011). Denmark was one of the first EU member states, along with Finland and Hungary, to receive a reasoned opinion from the European Court of Justice in March 2007 over restrictive practices in its betting market.

In September, 2011, the European Court of Justice ruled that Austria can bar foreign gaming firms from operating in the country on the basis that it is difficult for a member state to rely on checks made by the authorities of another member state using regulatory systems outside its control (Chee 2011). However, member states must provide evidence that monopolies guarantee a particularly high level of consumer protection to justify restrictive measures. It was made clear that gambling monopolies cannot be allowed if they seek to grow the gambling market, essentially requiring European governments to choose between revenue maximisation and the pursuit of high levels of consumer protection. In its ruling in the Austrian online gambling case Dickinger and Ömer (C-347/09), the court stated that "...*to be consistent with the objective of fighting crime and reducing opportunities for gambling, national legislation establishing a monopoly which allows the holder of the monopoly to follow an expansionist policy must genuinely be based on a finding that the crime and fraud linked to gaming are a problem in the Member State concerned, which could be remedied by expanding authorised regulated activities... policy of expanding games of chance characterised inter alia by the creation of new games and by the advertising of those games, such a policy cannot be regarded as being consistent unless the scale of unlawful activity is significant. The objective of protecting consumers from addiction to gambling is in principle difficult to reconcile with a policy of expanding games of chance... A distinction must therefore be drawn between a restrained commercial policy seeking only to capture or retain the existing market for the organisation with the monopoly, and an expansionist commercial policy whose aim is to expand the overall market for gaming activities*". Sigrid Ligné, Secretary General of the EGBA, commented that: "*Increasingly, the Member States of the EU are regulating the online gaming market on a multi license basis and that trend is also fostered by the European Commission pushing forward its Green Paper process on online gaming. This ruling signals yet again the urgent need for a comprehensive EU framework taking fully into account the cross border dimension of online gambling."*

A non-legislative resolution passed in October 2011 by the EU Internal Market Committee indicates the Parliament's position on the Green Paper that Member States should be free to maintain their own Internet gambling rules, but that there should be greater cooperation to counter the illegal market and protect children and vulnerable consumers (Internal Market and Consumer Protection Committee 2011). The resolution suggests introducing a licensing model to ensure that gambling providers meet the criteria imposed by Member States and that competition is fair and transparent. Stronger cooperation, such as an electronic linkage network and agreements between financial institutions, between regulatory bodies would enable common standards to be developed to take action against unlicensed gambling providers. Common standards for consumer protection were also cited as highly important.

Further reports, court cases and decisions are already underway and developments in Europe are likely to continue. The current situation of inter-jurisdictional inconsistency is creating ongoing problems for regulators, operators and consumers, although it may be difficult to develop common standards that are uniformly agreed upon. However, recent decisions indicate that there is an increased recognition of the importance of some level of cooperation. It is likely that the Internet gambling market in Europe will continue to expand and open as more consumer demand online gambling services and governments recognise the difficulties of prohibition and increase liberalisation.

United Kingdom

Following the implementation of the Gambling Act in 2007, the UK became a regulated free market for remote gambling operators. Internet gambling is regulated by the National Gambling Commission. The Gambling Commission was established under the Act and is an independent non-departmental public body responsible for issuing operating licenses to organisations and individuals who are providing facilities for online gambling. Online sports betting, horse race betting, betting exchanges, bingo, poker, and games of skill can be legally operated in the UK and played by British residents. UK-based sites and those on the White list (including Alderney, the Isle of Man, Antigua, Barbuda and Tasmania) are permitted to advertise directly to UK customers (Church-Sanders 2011). According to industry reports, there were 8.8 million unique UK visitors to online gambling sites each month in 2011, an increase of 28% from August 2009 (Church-Sanders 2011). The online gambling market in the UK is estimated at £1.48 billion (KPMG 2010).

By legalizing and regulating Internet gambling, the UK hoped to entice many offshore Internet gambling businesses back onshore and have them pay appropriate taxes in exchange for the privileges associated with being licensed (Atherton 2006).

However, the current system does not appear to be successful, resulting in offshore operators having a significant advantage over UK-based companies; for example paying around 1% tax as opposed to 15%, and attracting a significant proportion of the market share (O'Brien 2011). Consequently, the UK Government announced in July 2011 that offshore gambling operators selling or advertising online gambling products in the UK should be regulated and all remote gambling operators will be required to hold a Gambling Commission licence (Willems 2011). This policy change was reportedly based on an effort to improve the consumer protection offered to UK customers by regulating sites onshore, although the tax implications are also highly significant. Transitional licenses will be available to operators already licensed in trusted jurisdictions to minimise disruptions. Responses from legal and industry professionals indicate that an introduction of tax on profits and higher licensing and regulatory costs will likely be accepted by the industry, due to the significance of the UK online gambling market (Willems 2011). However, questions have been raised over how the regulations will be enforced and the implications for customers who may face higher costs.

Online gambling operators who are not compliant risk regulatory action by the Gambling Commission (Department for Culture, Media and Sport, Gambling Act 2005). The commission has a range of power that it may exercise following a review of the performance of licence holders against the terms of their license including:

- Issuing a warning to a license holder;
- Attaching an addition condition, removing or amending conditions to a licence;
- Suspending and revoking a license;
- Imposing a financial penalty following breach of a licence condition.

Alderney

Situated in the Channel Islands, off the French coast of Normandy, Alderney offers a well-regulated banking, insurance, and investment environment, with relatively low tax levels, minimal bureaucracy and has taken a pragmatic approach toward the regulation of the e-gambling industry (Wilsenach 2011). In 2000, the Alderney Gambling Control Commission (AGCC) was established to develop a regulatory framework for both electronic betting and interactive gambling. The AGCC seeks to meet 'world-class' standards that protect both the reputation of Alderney and attracts reputable operators who seek a comprehensive and tightly controlled regime (Wilsenach 2011). The main objectives of the AGCC are to ensure that (a) all forms of online gambling are conducted honestly and fairly, (b) the funding, management, and operation of e-gambling remains free from criminal influences and exploitation, (c) e-gambling activities are regulated and monitored so as to protect the public's interests, and (d) the potential harm that e-gaming and betting may cause to the public, individuals, and families is minimized. To achieve these aims, the Commission actively participates in other international regulatory bodies and seeks approval from three independent testing authorities.

Potential licence holders in Alderney must be a resident and its shareholders, key personnel and its sources of funding must satisfy the 'probity test'. Prior to launching an Internet gambling site, the licensee is required to obtain approval from the Commission for their Internet gambling equipment and control system submission. Following the granting of a licence, the Internet gambling system is tested by an independent authority and then accredited by the AGCC. Once a licensee is operational, regular and ad hoc inspections are conducted to ensure on-going compliance with the approved technical standards and internal control systems.

Germany

In 2008 Germany's State Treaty on Gambling was approved to reduce problem gambling resulting in online gambling through private providers being prohibited and advertising of gambling services banned (Gold Media 2010). Online gambling through state-owned monopolies is permitted in a regulatory model that is widely considered extremely restrictive (EGBA 2011). The European Union Court of Justice ruled in September 2010 that Germany's betting monopoly violates European laws because the German rules "do not limit games of chance in a consistent and systematic manner" to claim that they safeguarded gamblers from addiction, as opposed to merely protecting government revenues (Goodley 2011; White 2011). However, this ruling was overturned and the restrictive online betting licensing regime for sports betting was upheld in June, 2011, by the European Commission, which said the rules were in line with constitutional and EU law (Bennett 2011b). EU regulators are in talks with German officials, who are drafting new gambling rules and the European Commission has raised serious doubts over the compatibility of Germany's draft gambling law (Bennett 2011b).

According to the draft gambling laws, private gaming companies could bid for seven national betting licences from 2012, with the winners paying 16.7% tax on turnover (Goodley 2011). Bets would only be allowed on the outcome of games, not on events within the game such as half-time results and which players would score or in-run betting. On 18 July, 2011, the EU commission rejected the draft legislation for a new gambling regime with a request for further details and explanations to justify the draft with regard to the purpose, proportionality and coherence of its provisions (Ploeckl 2011). In September 2011, the German state of Schleswig-Holstein passed online gambling legislation that would allow online gambling licenses to be issued with an associated tax of 20% on gross profits (Kingsley 2011). Experts advise that the other German states would now be completed to open up their online gambling markets on more reasonable terms (Kingsley 2011). A spokesman for Germany-based Bwin.party said "There is still a long way to go. We remain confident that in the end the government will comply with European law and implement a commercially viable licensing regime to the benefit of all stakeholders" (Goodley 2011). Currently companies such as Bwin.party take unregulated bets from German residents that attract no tax.

According to industry consultants, German residents spend €800 million annually on offshore Internet gambling sites and are the second largest poker market in the world (Holliday 2011). In 2009 the share of the unregulated market was one-fifth, however if current trends persist, the illegal online gambling is expected to account for almost a third of the entire German gambling market (Gold Media 2010). Legal advisors have suggested that the protectionist policies are costing Germany €10 billion in revenues between 2012 and 2016 (Church-Sanders 2011). Concomitantly, state-run gambling providers have experienced a significant decline in revenue, despite overall growth in the online gambling market (Gold Media 2010). The continuation of the offshore gambling market could increase the incentive for change in the medium term; however, H2 Gambling Capital projected that a regulated market in Germany would capture only 7% of total Internet gambling activity in the territory should it proceed with the restrictive opening for sports betting proposed in April 2011 (Holliday 2011).

Italy

In 2007 regulation was passed in Italy making it legal for Italian citizens to gamble online (Church-Sanders 2011). It is estimated that 14,000 interactive and retail betting licences were awarded to private operators in early 2007. As the majority of the EU increases restrictions on online gambling, Italy acted in contrast by liberalizing its policies. As of May 2010, online gambling operators are no longer required to locate their companies and servers in Italy and licenses can be granted to domestic and European operators (Church-Sanders 2011). In addition to skill gaming, poker, casino games, fixed odds and pari-mutuel horse and sports betting can be conducted online. The Italian gambling market grew from €73 million (GGY) in 2007 to €781 million in 2010 and is expected to reach €1,674 million by 2015 due to the relative lack of competition (Holliday 2011). The promotion of local brands within the restrictive market appears to be successful as estimated indicate that over 85% of Italian player activity is expected within the regulated scheme by 2012 (Holliday 2011). Internet filters are used to block Italians from accessing sites not regulated within the country. The success of the Italian regulatory framework is attributed to the carefully balanced taxation system and levels of consumer protection offered (EGBA 2011). Analysis by PricewaterhouseCoopers (2011) predicts that Italy will soon overtake the UK as the largest legal online gambling market.

France

Historically, France has been monopolistic in gambling-related matters; however, in 2010, 17 online gambling licenses were issued to 19 different operators, ending the 471-year old gambling monopoly (Church-Sanders 2011). Internet gambling products permitted include horserace betting, poker, and sports wagering. Concurrently, the regulatory authority announced that it would consider legal action against unlicensed gambling operators allowing French citizens to use their websites and require French Internet service providers to block unregulated

gambling sites (Church-Sanders 2011). French Interactive Gambling GGW increased
from €200 million in 2008 to over €800 million in 2011 (Holliday 2011).

However, the French regulatory model has been criticised due to its excessively
high burdens on licensed gambling websites, notably with respect to taxes and technical requirements, and due to the limited product scope (EGBA 2011). For example, a study by Price Waterhouse Coopers shows that for an existing EU operator to
invest in France €8.7 million is required to cover the administrative and technical
costs for obtaining and maintaining the national license required (EGBA 2011).
Estimates indicate that up to 57–70% of the market is still offshore and existing
licensees may leave due to high taxation rates that limit player returns (EGBA 2011;
Holliday 2011). Speaking at a European iGaming conference, Emmanuel de Rohan
Chabot, CEO of horse racing betting specialist Zeturf, claimed that the high tax
rates have resulted in increased player expenditure; due to the maximum 85% return
to the player, customers are now spending an average of €100 a month rather than
the previous level of €60 (Church-Sanders 2011).

Sweden

State-owned gambling company Svenska Spel operates the country's licenses for
betting and gambling, including online gambling. In July 2010 the European Court
of Justice ruled that Sweden was entitled to restrict gambling to its state-owned
monopoly by banning other operators from advertising in the country (Church-
Sanders 2011). However, the Swedish laws are somewhat ineffective and 150 gambling companies are estimated to operate in Sweden (Church-Sanders 2011).

Svenska Spel's mandate is to meet Swedish demand for gambling in a safe and
responsible way free of private profit interests (Stymne 2008). Perhaps as a result of
the measures taken, Svenska Spel has reported a decline in net gaming revenue from
2009 to 2011 (Peppin 2011a). However, Svenska Spel had an increase in revenue in
the first quarter of 2011, compared to the same period in 2010 (EGBA 2011).
Although the state-owned monopoly is somewhat successful, many residents still
appear to be playing on offshore sites. In 2008 it was estimated that Svenska Spel's
poker site accounted for approximately 35% of the Internet poker market in Sweden
(Stymne 2008). There were 200,000 offshore Internet poker gamblers in 2007 and
105,000 Svenska Spel poker players. Of the Svenska Spel players, 65,000 started to
play poker at Svenska Spel and hadn't played Internet poker previously (and 35,000
still playing only at Svenska Spel) and 55,000 had started at other sites, and now
play either only at Svenska Spel or at both Svenska Spel and other sites.

The Netherlands

Legislation within the Netherlands prohibits residents from accessing online
gambling sites located outside the country (Wood and Williams 2007). In 2008,
the Netherlands Ministry of Justice rejected an online gambling bill that would

have allowed Holland Casino to provide casino games online and confirmed the introduction of measures that would impose criminal penalties on banks and credit card companies facilitating Dutch citizens gambling on foreign owned sites (Church-Sanders 2010). In October 2010, Dutch newspaper De Telegraaf, crediting "sources in The Hague", reported that the Dutch government was planning to go against previous policy and sell licenses or establish a competitive tender process (Church-Sanders 2011). The government is currently planning to establish a regulatory body to govern online gambling and legal online gambling is expected to be available from licensed operators from 2012 (PwC 2011). In the interim the government has announced that it is determined to eliminate unlicensed and illegal online gambling sites operating in the Dutch market (Balding 2011). The plan to liberalise the online gambling market has been criticised by the national slot machine organisation VAN, whose chairwoman, Anette Kok has stated that licenses should initially be provided only to operators with an established land-based business rather than opening the market with few restrictions ('Netherlands online plans' 2011).

Poland

In Poland the government has maintained its anti-gambling stance by releasing a draft amendment to its gambling legislation that confirms bans on all forms of online gambling, with the exception of sports betting (Balding 2011). This law advocates tough punitive measures against illegal or unauthorised online gambling operators and also those within Poland who facilitate or encourage online gambling at unauthorised sites. The European Commission has written to the Polish government over its failure to notify the EU of such gambling bans (Church-Sanders 2011). Despite the bans, Polish citizens regularly gamble on offshore sites and several large international sportsbooks offer Polish versions of their sites (Church-Sanders 2011).

Pacific

Australia

Internet gambling in Australia is regulated by the Interactive Gambling Act passed by the Federal Government in June 2001. Under this Act, individual states have the ability to formulate their own policies and legislation. This allows for the existence of a broad regulatory schema while still preserving the particular and individual economic policies and regulatory practices of each state and territory. Interactive gambling, including gambling through Internet, mobile applications and interactive television, is permitted for licensed wagering and lottery sites. Other online gambling sites (casino, slots, poker, bingo, etc.) are allowed to operate in Australia, but are not permitted to offer services or advertise to Australian residents.

In 2008, the High Court of Australia ruled unanimously in favour of allowing Western Australian residents to legally place bets with a licensed online betting exchange regulated in Tasmania (Monaghan 2008). The High Court decision effectively overturned state laws that restrict interstate gambling operators from competing within a state. Laws potentially under question include those regarding requirements for approval or fees to publish or use race fields, prohibitions and restrictions on advertisements, and restrictions on out-of-state bet types and product offerings. Laws restricting or prohibiting the location of out-of-state operator premises and equipment may also be implicated by the decision, particularly given the difficulty regulating telephone or Internet space. These changes may also potentially impact the value of licences and gambling tax rates. In 2010 the Productivity Commission published a comprehensive gambling inquiry report that issued the same recommendation as in 1999, that is, to liberalise and regulate Internet gambling. This recommendation was based on the conclusion that current policies are ineffective and do not support player protection or allow domestic operators to compete with offshore sites (Gainsbury 2010). This recommendation was rejected by the Federal Government (Gainsbury 2010).

Gambling is a popular entertainment activity in Australia, with total gambling expenditure of AUD$19.2 billion in 2010, or an average of $1500 per gambling adult (Productivity Commission 2010; Roy Morgan Research 2011). Industry estimates suggest that Australians spent AUD$968 million on offshore casino, poker and bingo sites in 2010 and spend $600 million per year on online sports gambling, including on legal and offshore sites (Global Betting and Gaming Consultants 2010). Gambling has become a heavily debated political issue in the past few years with heavy lobbying from industry groups, and those who support gambling reforms in an attempt to reduce related harms. Internet gambling regulation is currently under review with several inquiries, public hearings, and expert consultations held in 2010 and 2011 on this topic. In July, 2011, a spokesman for the Communications Minister, Stephen Conroy, stated that the government would conduct a review of the Interactive Gambling Act to examine the operation and the effectiveness of the current regulations ('Online Facebook betting' 2011). The review will consider international regulatory approaches to online gambling and their potential applicability to the Australian context in addition to the ability to improve harm minimisation measures for online gambling and the enforcement of existing prohibitions on certain types of gambling. Several research studies are also underway to further investigate the use of and impact of Internet gambling in Australia.

New Zealand

Exclusive operating rights for online race and sportsbooks have been granted to the Racing Board and online lotteries are operated by the Lotteries Commission (Monaghan 2008). All other forms of online gambling are prohibited in New Zealand and it is illegal to organize, manage or promote online gambling or to wager with offshore providers. In March, 2008 the New Zealand Government announced a decision to allow online sales of Lotto, Powerball, Strike, Big Wednesday, and Keno (Monaghan 2008). More recently, in July 2011, the National Lottery Commission announced plans to seek authorization to sell instant scratch tickets online in an effort to increase sales and profits (Petrolli 2011). Critics of online gambling in New Zealand have cited the impact of problem gambling in the community, and believe that the decision to allow Internet gambling will cause further problems because of the ease with which credit cards can be used to purchase tickets online.

Asia

The Asian market has been slower to develop due to difficulties in transferring money in and out of some countries, a general lack of reliable telecommunications infrastructure and widespread Internet access, lack of consistent policy and regulatory approval, and potential mistrust of electronic forms of gambling and monetary transfers (RSeConsulting 2006). Potential risks to the Asian online gambling industry include regulatory changes, increases in illegal gambling opportunities, and a potential rise in gambling taxes (Church-Sanders 2011). Internet gambling often operates through Internet cafes and is cash-based (Church-Sanders 2011). A positive development for online gambling is the emergence of a rapidly growing middle class with substantial and rising disposable income, particularly in China (Monaghan 2008).

China

Online gambling in China is almost completely prohibited by law and in 2009 China banned foreign investment into its online gambling industry and Internet gambling sites are targeted and blocked (Church-Sanders 2011). Since 2009, Chinese police have reportedly detained or arrested more than 7,360 people for establishing and running gambling websites, given fines of up to USD$735,000, prison terms ranging from 1 to 5 years, and frozen almost one billion yuan (USD$148 million), including non-Chinese residents (Beach 2009).

Online gambling is estimated to be widespread, and Casino City Online (2011) lists 180 Chinese-language sites that accept play from China. It is difficult to estimate the potential market size in China. Industry and academic estimates have valued the Chinese online gambling market at between US$12 billion and US$75 billion per year (Monaghan 2008). A survey conducted in 2011 by Credit Suisse asked 2,585 Chinese consumers what services they had utilised online in the past 6 months and 2% reported gambling (Stradbrooke 2011).

The Hong Kong Jockey Club (HKJC), a non-profit government body which administers and regulates horse racing and wagering, offers online lottery play, sports betting and horserace betting to Hong Kong and non-Hong Kong residents (Casino City Online 2011). The 2002 Gambling (Amendment) Ordinance prohibits

Hong Kong residents from engaging in online gambling with external operators outside of Hong Kong. Estimates suggest that 35% of the HKJC's bets on horse racing now come through its website or mobile devices, up from 22% in 2006 and these is a substantial proportion of bets being made with unauthorised on and offline bookmakers (Balfour 2011).

The government of Macau has authorized the Macau Jockey Club to offer horserace wagering products over the Internet (Casino City Online 2011). It has also authorized the Sociedade de Loterias e Apostas Mutuas de Macau to offer sports lottery products online. Foreign gambling providers are currently not permitted to offer remote services from Macau.

Philippines

The Philippines is the only country where online and mobile gambling is permitted, In the Philippines, the state-owned and controlled Philippines Amusement and Gaming Corporation is the sole authorized gambling operator (Casino City Online 2011). The company operates casinos, bingo, sports betting and betting exchanges online. In 2002, the government opened its Internet gaming industry to competition, including Internet cafes (PricewaterhouseCoopers, PWC 2010). Reports in 2011 indicate that police have been conducting raids against illegal online gambling operations run by organised crime that used a live dealer casino which online players at remote locations could see and bet via computers (Peppin 2011b).

Japan

Japan is estimated to have one of the world's largest online gambling markets, with more than ten million people wagering at online casinos, despite the fact that Internet gambling (other than lotteries and race wagering) is banned in Japan and there are no online Japanese casinos (KPMG 2010; PWC 2010). The Japanese Racing Association's interactive business is the largest interactive operator in the world, accounting for about a quarter of the non-addressable Internet gambling market (H2 Gambling Capital 2011). Reports indicate that the Japanese government are considering opening the land-based and online casino market, however this would be strictly controlled with protection for vulnerable groups (Church-Sanders 2011).

India

In India, online gambling is banned in Maharashtra, but there is no specific legislation in most other regions (PWC 2010). India currently operates an online lottery, however, the Indian government has been actively blocking gambling-related websites and ruled that gambling debts cannot be enforced, discouraging online gambling operators (Church-Sanders 2011). The Indian state of Sikkim is in the process of issuing online gambling licenses to target the Indian market ('Opportunities in Indian E-gaming market' 2011). Licenses would be valid for 5 years and allow casino gambling, poker and sports betting to be offered to Indian residents. In order to obtain a Sikkim licence, foreign companies must apply in a joint venture with a local company.

Internet penetration in India is very low at less than 7% of the population ('Opportunities in Indian E-gaming market' 2011). India's online gaming gross win was estimated to be worth US$70 million and may reach US$250 million by 2912 under partial state regulation (Church-Sanders 2011).

Africa

Internet uptake is growing strongly in Africa and about half the population have mobile phones demonstrating a desire for interactive technology, however, market penetration is still very low due to the lack of reliable infrastructure (Church-Sanders 2011). Mobile gambling is estimated to grow at last 20% per year from 2009 to 2014 in the Africa and Middle East regions (Church-Sanders 2011).

South Africa was expected to legalise online wagering several years ago, but have delayed the introduction of legislation to this effect (PWC 2010). In August 2010, courts forced foreign operators to stop accepting bets from South African citizens, and banks and credit card companies have blocked South Africans from using their credit cards on online gambling sites. One online operator appealed this decision and has continued to operate, although they may be forced to repay any profits if the appeal is unsuccessful (PWC 2010). New advertising rules introduced in October 2010 appeared to move towards prohibition of online gambling (Church-Sanders 2011). However, a review commission on the South African gambling industry and its regulation in August 2011 recommended that all forms of online gambling be made legal and regulated in recognition of the difficulties associated with prohibition (Merten 2011). The commission recommended that a limited number of licenses would initially be offered with advertising rights for licence holders and that banks would be involved in enforcing regulations. Industry consultants estimate that the online sports betting market in South Africa is worth £54.9 million and will grow to £77.7 million by 2010, although the effective target market is only around 10% of the total population who have access to the requisite technology (Church-Sanders 2011).

Central and South America

The online gambling industry in Central and South America has been obstructed by inconsistent or unclear regulatory environments in some of the major countries of the region (Church-Sanders 2011). A lack of necessary technological infrastructure and Internet penetration as well as poor online payment processing options will continue to delay the implementation of appropriate regulatory frameworks and market growth. However, the mobile industry is growing quickly, which will have a direct impact in the Internet gambling industry. Opportunities are beginning to emerge, with Panama expected to be the one of the most progressive jurisdictions, already permitting online sportsbooks and offering tax breaks for companies that cater to foreign customers to encourage an emphasis on offshore rather than domestic markets (Church-Sanders 2011).

Costa Rica has the largest gambling market in Latin America due to its favourable online gambling policies generating US$14.5 billion per year (Church-Sanders 2011). Internet gambling is legal in Chile, and online poker is very popular in this market (PWC 2010). Brazil has a strong base of regular Internet users and a cultural history of gambling, however Internet gambling is currently prohibited (KPMG 2010). Argentina is regarded as a key market for Internet gambling operators due to the popularity of sports betting and the substantial extent of Internet penetration (Church-Sanders 2011; Marrison 2011). Currently online gambling is banned in the national capital, Buenos Aires, but permitted by regional governments who have jointly issued three licenses for operators that are only allowed to accept local players (Church-Sanders 2011; Marrison 2011). Announcements have been made to indicate that Argentina will introduce national legislation by 2014 that would lead to legal online gambling in an effort to reduce play on offshore sites and raise funds to help fund football match broadcasts (Marrison 2011). Several large operators are already advertising in this region (Church-Sanders 2011; KPMG 2010). Although no online poker operators are legally operating within Argentina, poker is increasing in popularity with several poker television channels available, and prominent advertisements for online poker sites and free play sites, including a sponsorship deal with River Plate, one of the biggest and most emblematic football teams in Latin America (Marrison 2011).

Chapter 4
Characteristics of Internet Gamblers

Abstract Internet gambling is more than simply a technological medium through which to access traditional gambling products. It represents an entirely new mode and form of gambling that has changed the nature of gambling products and the way in which players use these. Online gambling has specific features that make it appealing and pose potential risks to players. In particular, it is highly accessible, convenient and affordable, offers a comfortable way for individuals to gamble anonymously in private on an immersive interface using electronic forms of money. Although many Internet gamblers appear to also engage in land-based gambling, Internet gamblers appear to be different from traditional gamblers and use online gambling for different reasons and in different ways. This chapter explores the differences between Internet and non-Internet gambling and gamblers. Research findings are presented to outline the demographic characteristics and breakdown of online gamblers and other related behaviours such as substance use. Details are provided of how online gamblers use the Internet for other purposes as well as their participation and behavioural patterns relating to online gambling. Motivations for online gambling and perceived advantages and disadvantages of this mode of access are discussed.

Keywords Internet gamblers • Online gambling • Demographics • Characteristics • Motivations • Advantages • Behaviour • Land-based gambling

Internet Gamblers

Much of what is currently known about online gamblers is primarily descriptive in nature and based upon convenience and self-selected samples, often recruited from a limited population (such as students at particular universities, players from one gambling site or forum); thus, the results may not be representative of the wider population of online gamblers. Results from the literature are described below, but caution is warranted in generalising the results too widely. Based on data taken from the 2007 UK Gambling Prevalence Survey, a regression analysis investigating the difference in socio-demographic factors between Internet gamblers and non-Internet gamblers found that the factors that most predicted Internet gambling were being male, younger, more highly educated, and drinking at least twice the daily recommended intake limits of alcohol (Griffiths et al. 2009a). Data analysis of a international sample of Internet (n = 1,954) and non-Internet (n = 5,967) gamblers recruited from an online gambling portal found that the variables that significantly predicted someone being an Internet gambler were: gambling on a greater number of formats, higher problem gambling severity score, male gender, tobacco use, being employed, younger age, more positive attitudes towards gambling, higher gambling expenditure, being single, alcohol use, illicit drug use, and higher household income (Wood and Williams 2011). Specific variables are discussed in more detail below; however, as online gambling participation grows, the market which is engaging in this form of gambling is also increasingly diversifying. This is clearly represented in discrepancies between studies and lack of a clear demographic group using the various forms of online gambling. Some preliminary research has been conducted in an effort to identify subgroups of Internet gamblers (Braverman and Shaffer 2010; Dragicevic et al. 2011; Wardle et al. 2011a). However, further research is needed to investigate how different segments of the population are engaging in online gambling and the impacts of this.

Gender

Internet gambling appears to be more popular among males than females (AGA 2006; Bernhard et al. 2007; eCOGRA 2007; Griffiths et al. 2009a; LaBrie et al. 2008; McBride and Derevensky 2009; LaBrie et al. 2008; Wood and Williams 2007, 2010). The UK Gambling Commission's ongoing survey for remote gambling has consistently found males to have about twice the rate of online gambling participation compared to females (Wardle et al. 2011a). However, there are a number of studies that suggest there may be a shift towards an increasing number of women gambling online, such that the number of women is equal to or greater than the number of men on Internet gambling sites (Corney and Davis 2010; McMillen and Woolley 2003; RSeconsulting 2006). Men and women typically engage in different types of online gambling; men prefer casino games, sports and race wagering and poker whereas women play more social games, such as bingo, that include chatrooms or chat functions (Broda et al. 2008; Church-Sanders 2010; eCOGRA 2007; Corney and Davis 2010; Wood and Williams 2011). Slot players are more likely to be women as these games can be played in short periods of time without interfering with other activities (Church-Sanders 2010).

Several studies have found women reporting that they would prefer to gamble online than in traditional venues as it was viewed as safer, less intimidating, anonymous, more fun and more tempting (Carpenter 2005; Griffiths 2001). The convenience of online gambling and ability to play for short periods of time, may also be appealing to women who take breaks from other responsibilities to play (Corney and Davis 2010), however these findings are preliminary and have not been fully investigated. Internet gambling provides an opportunity for operators to target women, who are not, for example, traditionally big users of betting shops (Ranade et al. 2006).

Many companies are targeting sites specifically at women; operators can use various targeting methods such as the names of sites, for example, www.ladycasino. com, www.cameocasino.com, and seek to appeal to women by using pink graphics, and having non-gambling pages such 'Gambling horoscopes' and 'Hunk of the month'. Advertisements for Paddy Power's bingo site appeared to target women by depicting a man with a naked chest attempting to breastfeed a baby with the slogan, 'Where have all the women gone?'(this advertisement received many complains and was subsequently deemed offensive and rejected by sensors). In addition, some sites are targeting women by offering novelty bets, on celebrities and pop culture (Ranade et al. 2006). In contrast, the majority of sites target young men, in particular sports fans, who are viewed as an ideal market that is already interested in the outcomes of games (Lamontet al. 2011). Advertisements often depict scantily clad women, provocative statements, and contain themes of money, sex, power, and enhanced social status as a result of online gambling (Monaghan et al. 2009; Derevensky et al. 2010). The relative ease at which an online gambling site can be created and modified means that operators can create different sites, or skins, with varying graphics, names, and themes to appeal to different groups, using the same games and products. This is a distinct advantage of Internet gambling as compared to land-based gambling in terms of customer recruitment and satisfaction.

Age

Internet gamblers are most likely to be less than 40 years of age (American Gaming Association 2006; Bernhard et al. 2007; LaBrie et al. 2008; McBride and Derevensky 2009; Ladd and Petry 2002; Wood and Williams 2007, 2010; Woodruff and Gregory 2005), although some research suggests that the most likely age bracket is 35–54 years (Woolley 2003; Levine 2010). The 2007 UK gambling prevalence survey found that Internet gamblers were more likely to be aged 34 years and younger (55%) and only 21% were older than 45 years, as compared to non-Internet gamblers, who were more likely to be aged 45–64 (Griffiths et al. 2009a). Online gambling also appears to be more prevalent amongst youth and young adults than the general adult population (Dowling et al. 2010; Griffiths and Barnes 2008; Griffiths et al. 2009a; McBride and Derevensky 2009; Olason et al. 2011; Wood and Williams 2010).

Age may also be related to type of online gambling; an Australian survey reported that younger adults were more likely to wager on sports using the Internet, while older adults were more likely to be using premium text-messaging to transfer funds (Phillips and Blaszczynski 2010). Similarly, Woolley (2003) found that 35–54 was the most common age group among sports and horse race bettors in Australia and LaBrie et al. (2007) found the average age of European sports bettors to be

31 (SD = 10). eCOGRA (2007) found the most common age group for online poker players to be 26–35 who were more likely to be males, and that online casino players were likely to be 46–55 and female, indicating that this mode of gambling appeals to different segments of the population.

Socio-Demographic Characteristics

In general, Internet gamblers are more likely to be better educated than non-Internet gamblers, work fulltime in managerial or professional occupations or be students and earn above-average salaries (AGA 2006; Bernhard et al. 2007; Griffiths et al. 2009a; Jiménez-Murcia et al. 2011; Levine 2010; McBride and Derevensky 2009; Jiménez-Murcia et al. 2011; Volberg et al. 2006; Wood and Williams 2007, 2011; Woodruff and Gregory 2005; Woolley 2003). In the UK, the prevalence of Internet gambling is higher among those with a degree, whereas the prevalence of non-Internet gambling was lowest among this group (Griffiths et al. 2009a). In the general UK population, non-Internet gamblers were more likely to be aged 35 and over, have no educational qualifications and be from a routine or manual household (Griffiths et al. 2009a). These socio-demographic characteristics of Internet gamblers are not surprising given the required technology ownership, basic technological ability and reliable access to the Internet that is required to gamble online.

Fewer reliable details are available on other socio-demographic characteristics of Internet gamblers. Furthermore, these details are much harder to access and understand due to the limited interactions that online gambling operators have with customers. Online gambling operators typically know a customer's age, gender, address, banking details and potentially credit history, and even IP address. With increased customer engagement through other channels, particularly social networking and in some cases loyalty programs, online gambling operators can access further details about their customer to facilitate a greater understanding of players. Some research has investigated demographic characteristics of online gambling, although results are not representative of Internet gamblers generally. In a large international sample of gamblers, compared to non-Internet gamblers, Internet gamblers were less likely to be married (Wood and Williams 2011). This is inconsistent with previous findings that Internet gamblers are more likely to be married (Wood and Williams 2007; Woodruff and Gregory 2005). Wood and Williams (2007) also found that 53% of Internet gamblers described themselves as religious people and were most likely to be Christian. The majority of this sample was from the US, which may account for some of the results.

Health and Substance Use

Several studies have investigated whether Internet gamblers are more likely to use alcohol, tobacco and other drugs than non-online gamblers in an effort to determine whether Internet gamblers are at greater risk of addictions. In a survey of 563 online gamblers, 45% of respondents reported consuming alcohol while gambling online, 33% reported using tobacco, 9% reported using marijuana or hashish, and 4% reported using other illicit drugs (McBride and Derevensky 2009). Other reports indicate that a large proportion of poker players use drugs including marijuana, cocaine, amphetamines, Valium, and other prescription medications as well as substances including caffeine, energy drinks and guarana to help them focus and concentrate as well as to calm nerves and improve memory. A significant proportion of Internet gamblers appear to use drugs to stay awake during extended gambling sessions, which may have serious negative consequences in terms of disrupted sleep and eating patterns and overall mental and physical health. An online survey of Internet gamblers in which participants were recruited from online gambling sites found that 12.3% of the sample (N = 1,920) described themselves as 'disabled' (Wood and Williams 2007). This may meant that those with limited mobility may gravitate to Internet gambling although it may also represent the bias of the self-selected sample of individuals willing to complete online questionnaires.

Several large studies have attempted to compare the substance use and health of Internet and non-Internet gamblers. The 2007 UK prevalence survey found that smoking status was associated with both gambling on the Internet and offline forms and Internet gamblers (64%) were significantly less likely to smoke than non-Internet gamblers (73%; Griffiths et al. 2009a). However, alcohol intake was related to past year Internet gambling as this group were significantly more likely to drink more heavily than non-Internet gamblers. No significant differences were found in the self-reported health status for Internet and non-Internet gamblers. Similarly, the majority of Internet gamblers in a Canadian sample of gamblers reported using alcohol when gambling, as compared to a minority of non-Internet gamblers (Wood and Williams 2010). However, in a large sample of international gamblers, no major differences were found in the alcohol use of Internet versus non-Internet gamblers (Wood and Williams 2010). When the samples were combined, Internet gamblers reportedly had higher rate of substance abuse or dependence (13.0% vs. 11.5%), as well as a higher rate of addictions in other areas (10.4% vs. 6.7%), than non-Internet gamblers (Wood and Williams 2011). Internet gamblers were more likely to use drugs while gambling (10.8%) as compared to non-Internet (3.7%) gamblers, and occasional and frequent use of drugs was reportedly much more common amongst Internet gamblers. No differences have been reported in past year serious mental health problems or physical disabilities between Internet and non-Internet gamblers.

As demonstrated, mixed results have been found and levels of alcohol, drug and smoking among Internet gamblers as a whole is still unclear. However, it is likely that there is a subgroup of Internet gamblers that gravitate towards this form due to the ability to drink alcohol, smoke and use drugs, which is often restricted in gambling venues, depending on jurisdictional regulation. Due to the relative lack of potential interruptions, excessive alcohol or drug use during online gambling may be associated with significant negative consequences.

General Internet Use

Not surprisingly, Woodruff and Gregory (2005) reported that accessibility to the Internet was related to Internet gambling. Those gambling on the Internet were more likely to have Internet access at home and at work and spent more time online in general than non-Internet gamblers. A survey of Nevada residents found that participants reported a lack of access or knowledge of how to use the Internet were obstacles that kept them from wagering online (Bernhard et al. 2007). However, although time spent online may predict future online gambling, neither location nor availability to Internet access was reported by gamblers to be a significant indicator of past or predicted future Internet gambling intentions (Woodruff and Gregory 2005). Internet gamblers reported they were more "likely to experiment", more "likely to try new products and ideas", and "liked variety" significantly more than non-Internet gamblers. However, as this study was conducted in the earlier years of online gambling, these participants may represent 'early adopters' and online gambling may be more accepted and a mainstream activity now. Nonetheless, online gamblers appear to be computer and Internet literate and generally use the Internet for multiple activities including communication, retrieving information and conducting business and banking, as well as purchasing products and services (American Gaming Association 2006; Wood and Williams 2007; Woodruff and Gregory 2005; Woolley 2003). An Australian survey found that factors that were related to use of interactive services included a tendency to respond impulsively, an interest in gambling, preoccupation with technology for entertainment and an interest in competitions (Phillips and Blaszczynski 2010).

Use of Internet Gambling Sites

Internet gamblers may bet from a variety of locations including work and through mobile devices, but betting from home appears to be by far the most common way of engaging with this form of gambling (eCOGRA 2007; McBride and Derevensky 2009; McMillen 2004; Wood and Williams 2007, 2010; Woodruff and Gregory 2005). As most Internet gamblers are employed, online gambling typically occurs in the evening (Wood and Williams 2010). A large survey of international internet gamblers reported that the majority of players gamble online between 6 pm and midnight (64%), although some players gamble during the afternoon (16%; Wood and Williams 2010). Only 10% of participants reported typically playing between midnight and 6 am, suggesting a minority may experience disrupted sleep patterns associated with Internet gambling. Surveys of participants from Australian wagering and casino-sites found that approximately 20% of participants reported gambling online with others and a larger proportion of females than males wagered online with their spouse (McMillen 2004).

Research findings suggest that most players utilise more than one gambling site and hold multiple accounts (McBride and Derevensky 2009; Wood and Williams

2010; Woolley 2003). Australian research reported that online wagerers were more likely than casino gamblers to have just one account, although the number of players with just one account declined over the 2 year period of the study (McMillen 2004), which itself was conducted some time ago suggesting that this trend may have continued. Responses to a survey on the state-owned Swedish Internet gambling site indicated that 62% of participants did not gamble online with anyone else but Svenska Spel (Griffiths et al. 2009b), although these participants were self-selected and may have been a biased sample.

The extent to which Internet gamblers engage in multiple forms of online gambling is difficult to estimate given the lack of detail in most prevalence studies and the difficulty tracking players across multiple gambling accounts. A survey of Internet gamblers revealed that participants appeared to involve themselves in a variety of online games, although some were tried once or twice (Wood and Williams 2007). Some online gambling sites offer multiple gambling options, for example, sports books may also include poker and casino games. Data regarding customers of one large European sportsbook (bwin) showed that the majority of account holders engaged primarily in sports gambling (LaBrie et al. 2008). Of 48,114 subscribers that opened an account in February 2005, 18% played casino games, although only 9% played casino games on more than 3 days. Similarly, of the original sample, only 9% played poker on the site, and 7% played poker for more than 3 days (LaPlante et al. 2008). It is unknown how many players had accounts with other operators, which limits the conclusions that can be drawn about this sample of online gamblers. However, these findings suggest that individuals may be selective in the types of online gambling forms that they play.

It is highly likely that online gamblers hold account with multiple sites given the high level of competition between sites and efforts placed on customer acquisition and retention by operators. Online gamblers are likely to 'shop around' for the most competitive odds and bonuses, including payback rates for customers. More involved bettors, including professional and semi-professional sports and race wagerers, are likely to spend more time looking for the best odds, as compared to recreational gamblers, who may keep accounts open and place bets with operators that provide them with ongoing bonuses. Operators that offer multiple types of gambling, such as side casino games on wagering sites and poker on casino and wagering sites, may offer a simple solution for players that prefer to limit the number of accounts that they open. This is likely to be an important area for future research, and one that is of significant interest to online gambling operators.

Overall Gambling Involvement

Internet gamblers typically engage in other forms of gambling in addition to online play (Griffiths et al. 2009a; South Australian Centre for Economic Studies 2008; Wood and Williams 2011), suggesting online play is one mode used, but not necessarily the preferred form of gambling for all Internet gamblers. Internet gamblers appear to be more involved gamblers generally as compared to non-Internet gamblers. Research has found that Internet gamblers typically have greater involvement in all types of gambling relative to non-Internet gamblers (AGA 2006; Gainsbury and Blaszczynski 2011b; Griffiths et al. 2009a; Volberg et al. 2006; Wood and Williams 2011). For example, findings from the 2007 UK prevalence survey indicated that Internet gamblers are more active bettors with 75% of those who gambled on eight or more activities being Internet gamblers and only 3% of Internet gamblers reporting gambling on just two activities (Griffiths et al. 2009a). Similarly, in an international sample, Internet gamblers reported involvement with an average of 4.1 different forms of gambling, versus an average of only 2.6 for non-Internet gamblers (Wood and Williams 2011).

The use of non-Internet gambling sites in addition to online gambling sites is of interest to many stakeholders for various reasons. Regulators and policy makers, as well as operators, are interested in the potential transition from land-based gambling to online forms. For some types of gambling, particularly betting and lottery, this transition is relatively straightforward as the same product is being offered, only the means of placing bets is different. In most cases, the same operator provides the different access modes. Many poker players engage in online and offline forms, and online poker does resemble land-based play in many ways and has the advantage of allowing more rapid play of multiple hands, against a larger cohort of players. Online casino games are also very similar to land-based games. As presented above, there is some evidence that online gamblers have adopted this mode of gambling and have not previously engaged in land-based gambling, either due to a lack of interest, lack of access or dislike for venues. It is also highly likely that some gamblers switch to Internet gambling in preference to land-based forms, for the convenience and accessibility as well as better odds and rates offered to players. This is an understudied area, although it is very important in understanding the impact of online gambling and the manner in which this mode is adopted by various segments of the population. It also has significant implications in relation to the causality of, continuance and incidence of problem gambling.

Expenditure, Time, and Patterns of Play

There is relatively little comprehensive information about global online gambling behaviour due to a lack of a single data source. Online gambling operators can provide data on how customers use each site, however, due to the numerous accounts held by online players, it is difficult to track behaviour across sites. Similarly, research is limited as it is typically based on self-report from a non-representative sample, or analysis of data from a single gambling operator. Understanding global patterns of play is an important area for future research.

Nonetheless, some research has been conducted to investigate patterns of online gambling Internet gamblers appear to spend more gambling per month than non-Internet gamblers (Gainsbury and Blaszczynski 2011b; Wood and Williams 2011).

In an international sample, Internet gamblers reported a net monthly expenditure of –US$195.14 compared to -US$70.93 spent by non-Internet gamblers, just over a third of what Internet gamblers spent (Wood and Williams 2010). The median net monthly expenditure for the Internet gamblers was –US$80.00, which is more than four times the median expenditure of –US$19.26 reported by the non-Internet gamblers. However, online gambling expenditure still appears to occur at relatively low levels. A survey conducted by eCOGRA found that 18% of Internet casino players wagered between $30–$60 per session, and online poker players most commonly (61%) played minimum stake levels of $0.50–$2.00 (eCOGRA 2007). An online survey of 563 Internet gamblers reported that the majority of players (55%) wagered less than CAD$25 per session, although 49% of participants reported wagering over $1,000 in a single Internet gambling session (McBride and Derevensky 2009), indicating high levels of variability both between players and between sessions of play. High stakes players, including professional and semi-professional online gamblers, are likely to have significantly higher expenditure for online gambling, although these players may be expected to lose a significantly lower proportion of their bets, particularly when comps and paybacks are included in calculations. Online gambling operators are likely to recognise large players and have special arrangements that limit the losses of these customers.

Surveys of Internet gamblers indicate that online gambling sessions typically last less than 2 h and very brief sessions of play also possible and common (McBride and Derevensky 2009; Wood and Williams 2007, 2010; Woolley 2003). Within eCOGRA's (2007) study, participants reporting playing on average 2–3 times per week for 1–2 h per session and have played for 2–3 years. This is consistent with findings by Wood and Williams (2007), who reported that the average weekly amount of time invested in online gambling was 5 h, with a media of 2 h, although 4.1% claimed to gamble in excess of 20 h per week.

Surveys of participants from Australian wagering and casino-sites found that players were roughly split with around half reporting spending more than 2 h in a typical online gambling session, and half spent less than 1 h per week (McMillen 2004), indicating that online gamblers are heterogeneous and have different levels of involvement.

Internet gambling is typically a solitary activity, although online gamblers may also gamble online with friends and family members (McBride and Derevensky 2009; McMillen 2004). In one Australian study, solitary online bettors spent more time gambling online than people who gamble in the company of others, although solitary casino players spend less time than those gambling with others (McMillen 2004), this may indicate differences between forms of online gambling and the types of people who play these. Overall, people who gamble alone spent more money than those who gamble with others and males tended to spend higher amounts than females, which was more marked with wagering than casino gambling (McMillen 2004).

Analysis of betting patterns amongst a large sample of 40,499 online sports bettors who opened an account with a European sports-book site (bwin) over an 8 month period found that the vast majority of sports bettors and casino game players appeared to have well controlled and moderated online betting behaviour (LaBrie et al. 2007, 2008). Amongst sports bettors, the typical pattern of gambling behaviour incurred a loss of 29% of the amount wagered (LaBrie et al. 2007). While the majority of individuals made bets of moderate proportions (less than €5), the top 2–3% of bettors wagered approximately €10,000 during the 8 month period. Analyses of playing behaviour found that in general individual gambling activity levels were moderate, as evidenced by analysis of time (people were active less than ½ of the time, despite infinite access), activity (most placed less than 4 bets/day during active periods) and expenditures (placing bets less than €5) (LaBrie et al. 2007). Furthermore, customers appeared to moderate their behaviour based upon previous wins and losses. As percent of loss increased, duration of play, total number of bets, bets per day, Euros per bet, and total wagers all decreased.

Further analyses also revealed that the population of online sports wagerers adapted to new subscription services, as evidenced by quickly developing declines in participation, number of bets, and size of stakes (LaPlante et al. 2008). Analysis revealed that a small proportion of bettors exhibited highly involved behaviour and these individuals had increasing stakes and bets for live-action betting over time (LaBrie et al. 2007). As these findings are based on a cohort recruited from a single European sports wagering site, they may not be generalisable to all Internet gamblers.

Use of casino games was also examined amongst this cohort and findings suggested that the majority of play was modest (LaBrie et al. 2008). The typical daily cost of online gambling was greater than for sports wagering amongst the same cohort, with a median bet of €6.5 per day, which is larger than the typical €1.2 daily cost of fixed-odds betting and the €0.8 typical daily cost for live action bets. However, the casino game gamblers played less frequently than the sports bettors, around twice a month, compared to about seven times a month for the sports bettors. Casino game bettors also incurred larger losses at each gambling session compared to sports bettors. As with the sports bettors, wagering decreased as losses increased and a subgroup of 5% of casino game players were more heavily involved than the majority of the sample, playing more frequently and with bets four times the size of the majority of players.

Analysis of behavioural data of 4,459 poker players on the same European sports wagering site (bwin) found that the vast majority of players played moderately and bought a median of €12 worth of chips at each of two poker sessions per week over a period of 6 months (LaPlante et al. 2009). These players appeared to moderate their behaviour based on wins and losses, where losses discouraged ongoing play and winning encouraged continued play. A smaller proportion (approximately 5%), were more involved and bough a median of €89 worth of chips at each of 10 poker sessions per week over 18 months. These players did not moderate their behaviours in response to losses, although they did appear to reduce the amount wagered as their losses increased proportionally. As with both sample above, these observations were based on customers of a sports wagering site, so they may not be representative of poker players more generally, and the individuals may also play on other sites and engage in other forms of online gambling.

Further research of Internet gambling behaviour has been conducted using player account data obtained from GTECH G2, and Internet gambling software provider for lotteries and casino gambling operators (Dragicevic et al. 2011). Analysis of 546 active online casino game (including roulette, slots, table games, and video poker) provides evidence of different gambling patterns amongst players. Four clusters of players were identified; 15% of the players demonstrated a higher frequency of gambling (4.35 bets per day), and increased frequency over time; 77% of players gambled moderately, at lower frequency than other groups and lost the least amount of money, although had a reasonably high variation in bet size; 1% of players showed high variability in the amounts bet, gambled frequently and intensively and lost the most money; and 5.7% of players demonstrated highly intensive betting patterns and had the highest variation in bet sizes. The most intensive gamblers, who also lost substantial amounts of money, spent the majority of their time gambling on slot games, followed by roulette. Slot games were also the most popular amongst those who gambled more frequently as compared to the entire cohort. The more moderate players engaged in all types of casino games, with table games being the most popular. This may indicate a preference for slot games amongst more involved players who may be at risk for experiencing gambling problems.

Motivations for Internet Gambling

Internet gambling has certain features that differentiate it from traditional land-based gambling and play a role in motivations for engaging in this form of gambling. However, as mentioned above, there is little evidence regarding the pathways of transition to Internet gambling from land-based gambling, or adoption of Internet gambling. Although Internet gambling participation rates have increased internationally, gambling participation rates overall do not appear to have increased, suggesting that Internet gamblers may have adopted this form in addition to or instead of other forms of gambling. There is also some evidence that individuals are gambling online, who would not gamble on land-based forms (Corney and Davis 2010; Griffiths 2001; McCormack and Griffiths 2011; Wood, Williams et al. 2007).

Trust in an Internet gambling operator is a crucial factor in determining whether an individual is willing to gamble online. Numerous studies in ecommerce suggest that an Internet site's ability to create trust among customers is one of the most important elements in facilitating ongoing usage and has long term consequences in terms of customer loyalty and retention (Fang et al. 2007; Johnson and Hult 2008; Reichheld and Schefter 2000; Urban et al. 1999). This is further demonstrated by the willingness of players to return to PokerStars following the US indictments; customer numbers have returned to previous levels due to the ability of the site to refund its player's money (Kimber 2011). This is a minimum requirement, on which additional motivations can be built to lead to ongoing Internet gambling.

The most obvious attributes of Internet gambling are the greater convenience, comfort and ease of access, which are repeatedly cited as the primary reason for gambling online in multiple studies (AGA 2006; Griffiths and Barnes 2008; Wood, Williams et al. 2007). This is confirmed by a survey of Nevada residents, in which those who had recently moved to the state indicated that online gambling became less appealing than it was when they lived in an area without significant access to traditional gambling outlets (Bernhard et al. 2007).

An online survey of an international sample of Internet gamblers reported that convenience was a key advantage of online gambling (Wood and Williams 2010). The 24-h availability (57%) and not having to drive or leave the house (51%) were the two most popular advantages stated as compared to land-based gambling. Interestingly, higher payout rates were only cited by 8% of the sample, indicating that this was not a significant advantage for most participants.

Amongst a small sample of British university online gamblers reasons given for online gambling were flexibility of use, 24 h availability, peer and familial influences, large variety of gambling choices, advertising, anonymity, and demo games (Griffiths and Barnes 2008). In the AGA (2006) study, participants reported gambling online as it was fun, exciting and entertaining, offered the opportunity to win money, and for anonymity and privacy. Youth (aged 12–24) described gambling online to relieve boredom and for excitement (McBride 2006). Other desirable features of online gambling reported include an aversion to the atmosphere and clientele of land-based venues, a preference for the pace and nature of online gameplay and the potential for higher wins and lower overall expenditures when gambling online (Wood, Williams et al. 2007). The ability to pretend to be the opposite sex has also been cited as a significant advantage, with women pretending to be males to be taken more seriously and for a greater sense of security, and males pretending to be females for supposed tactical advantages (Griffiths 2003, 2006).

Several qualitative studies in which Internet and non-Internet gamblers have been interviewed provide further details on motivation for gambling online. A study by Parke and Griffiths (2001) found that Internet gamblers were more likely to be financially stable and gamble within a set budget, gambled less for emotional reasons, reported fewer physiological effects (e.g., increased heart rate), and appeared to be more competitive than non-Internet gamblers. Traditional gamblers expressed a desire to gamble online for convenience, the improved facilities and tax-free betting. However, the barriers to doing so included having to obtain valid credit or debit cards and the inability to collect winnings in cash, thus reducing the enjoyment of wins. In a comparison of US gamblers, Cotte and Latour (2009) found that Internet gamblers preferred to gamble alone or with family, online gambling was a safer and less arousing environment, online gamblers reported greater perceptions of control over time and money spent, although online gamblers may spend more time gambling and alter their work and family schedule to fit around this activity.

A qualitative study interviewed 29 participants including online, offline and non-gamblers aged 19–58 years to examine motivating and inhibiting factors for gambling online (McCormack and Griffiths 2010). Results identified that the major motivator for gambling online was that it provided a greater opportunity to gamble. Sub themes identified included the convenience, value for money, greater variety of games and anonymity. Convenience was related to the lack of travel time and time constraints as online gambling could be made to structure around activities as home, or be used during spare time. Value for money reflected the more competitive prices and promotional offers typically offered online including bonus start-up credit, low stakes possible options, and the ability to play for free until confidence is established. Greater online variety included the ability to play multiple poker games simultaneously, and anonymity reduced social anxiety and stigma for gamblers, including females who reported being intimidated in venues. However, as the recruitment source was not specified it is difficult to determine how representative the views expressed are.

Perceived Disadvantages of Internet Gambling

There still remains some level of mistrust and cynicism amongst consumers regarding online gambling, with security concerns and legitimacy cited as the primary reasons for not playing online (Ipsos Reid 2005; Woodruff and Gregory 2005). A study by the AGA (2006) suggests 55% of a sample of online gamblers believe that online casinos cheat players. Similarly, in a comparison of Internet and non-Internet gamblers (Woodruff and Gregory 2005), belief about trusting the security of payment for Internet winnings was found to be a significant predictor of Internet gambling behaviour. Individuals who were non-Internet gamblers were found to have less trust in a fair payment system. Other concerns focused upon the trustworthiness of the site itself have been frequently raised.

When asked about the disadvantages of gambling online, Internet gamblers most frequently identified issues related to fairness and security (Wood and Williams 2010). The most commonly identified disadvantage was the difficulty in verifying the fairness of games (36%), followed be worrying about monetary deposits being safe and having wins paid in a timely fashion (25%). Some participants were worried about illegality of online gambling, the poorer social atmosphere and game experience (all 18–19%). Some players appeared concerned with the potential negative consequences of online gambling reporting that it was easier to spend more money online (19%), too convenient (16%) and more addictive (12%).

In a large-scale survey of international Internet gamblers, over one-third of respondents claimed to have had a dispute at some point with an operator, with less than half of these saying it had been successfully resolved (eCOGRA 2007). In the first 6 months of 2011, independent player protection organisation eCOGRA reported a total of 475 disputes submitted online, with the number of valid disputes resolved in favour of the player dropping to 40%, down 3% on the same period in 2010 ('Fall in disputes' 2011). The valid and legitimate complaints featured cash-in problems (41%), bonus issues (23%), and locked accounts (21%) as the main disputes. Regardless of whether attitudes are based on actual problems with the fairness and integrity of sites or a misunderstanding of the consumer protection measures offered, consumer confidence and trust in a site is vital to success in terms of customer loyalty and retention (Fang et al. 2007; Johnson and Hult 2008;

Reichheld and Schefter 2000; Urban et al. 1999). Improving levels of confidence in online gambling sites is expected to increase participation and spending among current Internet gamblers (Jolley et al. 2006; Toce-Gerstein and Gerstein 2007) and may enhance trust among non-Internet gamblers (Ipsos Reid 2005; Woodruff and Gregory 2005).

Concerns regarding fair play practices are reasonable as there are numerous examples of online gambling sites not paying winnings, cheating players with unfair games or stealing player deposits (Games and Casino 2006; McMullan and Rege 2010). Instances have been reported of employees of large online gambling sites cheating players, and selling customer identities and credit card details (McMullan and Rege 2010).Due to the highly competitive market, a number of Internet gambling operators, including large, well regarded companies, have declared bankruptcy and closed sites leaving customer accounts unpaid (Barker 2007). For example, recent prosecutorial actions against Absolute Poker and Ultimatebet by the US authorities have resulted in these sites declaring bankruptcy, leaving players with little recourse in accessing funds deposited in accounts ('DoJ attack' 2011). Other unscrupulous gambling operators set up Internet gambling sites for the sole purpose of stealing customer's money and identity data (McMullan and Rege 2010). Security breaches are damaging to the reputation of specific sites and to the entire industry and operators and regulators should take steps to increase customer protection and consumer trust.

The major inhibiting factor that emerged from interviews with 29 participants as a reason for not gambling online was the reduced authenticity of gambling online (McCormack and Griffiths 2010). Sub-themes included the reduced realism, the asocial nature of the Internet, the use of electronic money, and concerns about the safety of online gambling sites. The reduced realism of online play was related to the lack of non-verbal communication between poker players, the use of electronic money rather than cash for wagers and winnings, and playing against 'a computer', which all appeared to reduce the enjoyment of gambling. Although some online gamblers reported using the social features of gambling websites to chat about the game, learn strategies and congratulate other players, nearly a third of offline gamblers reported that they did not gamble online as it was viewed as antisocial. The majority of gamblers indicated that electronic money did not seem as real and there was a perception that it was more easily spent than cash. Finally, a number of gamblers were unsure about the safety of Internet gambling, which is consistent with previous research (AGA 2006; Ipsos Reid 2005).

Chapter 5
Risks Associated with Internet Gambling

Abstract The anonymous nature of Internet gambling and lack of rigorous regulation make online gamblers susceptible to specific risks. Disputes with online gambling sites can occur and examples are discussed including unfair games, player deposits and winnings not being returned, identity theft, and cheating by players. Internet gambling sites can be used for criminal purposes and operators and regulators must take measures to protect players and detect any illegal activity. Potential cheating includes inside information being used to set odds and cheating by players, officials or other involved individuals to win bets. Such cheating can take advantage of players and online sites and is increasingly monitored. This chapter outlines ways in which online gambling sites and operators can act to reduce risks to players and demonstrate the safety and security of their sites as well as ways in which players can minimize their own risks.

Keywords Fraud • Money laundering • Cheating • Online gambling • Internet gambling • Criminal activity • Hacking • Customer protection • Risks

Although many Internet gambling sites are licensed and abide by relatively stringent requirements for customer protection, the borderless and online nature of the activity poses substantial risks for customers. The EU Commission calculated that there are more than 12,500 sites in Europe operating without a license of any sort (European Commission 2011a). These sites are therefore not checked by any sort of body or authority and are free to cheat players, steal deposits and act in generally in a fraudulent and deceptive manner. It is important for players to be aware of this activity and take steps to protect themselves and for regulators to educate consumers about the risks of unregulated sites and take actions to reduce the extent to which these operators can offer products to residents.

There are numerous examples of online gambling sites not paying winnings, cheating players with unfair games or stealing player deposits (Games and Casino 2006). In 2008, players at two large online poker sites, Absolute Poker and Ultimate

Bet, found that employees had cheated players out of more than US$23 million by using insider information and software codes to access player's private accounts (McMullan and Rege 2010). In addition to money, identity theft is a potential concern in relation to Internet gambling. Examples include a CD containing the personal details of 17,000 player accounts at the German lottery operator Süddeutsche Klassenlotterie being sold to call centres. In another example, a sports betting site, BetOnSports, was hacked with the help of an insider, with identifying details, credit card and bank account numbers stolen and subsequently used internationally for illegal activities (McMullan and Rege 2010). In March and April 2010, Betfair's systems were allegedly infiltrated in an attack thought to originate in Cambodia, and payment card details of about 2.3 million customers were allegedly stolen in addition to usernames with encrypted security questions, addresses and bank account details ('Betfair kept massive card data theft quiet' 2011). The security breach was not discovered until May 2011 and customers were not informed.

Another type of risk for consumers is the possibility of online gambling sites declaring bankruptcy and not returning player deposits. Due to the highly competitive market, a number of Internet gambling operators, including large, well regarded companies, have declared bankruptcy and closed sites leaving customer accounts unpaid (Barker 2007).

Customers also face significant risks playing on sites that are not legally operating in the jurisdiction in which they are located. Most recently, following the indictments brought against several large poker sites operating in the US, many US and Canadian customers lost their account deposits. A class-action lawsuit has been launched by Canadian players against Full Tilt Poker in an effort to recover between CAD$5 million and CAD$10 million in player accounts (Moore 2011). It is also estimated that US players are missing as much as USD$150 million as a result of Full Tilt's practice of improperly crediting player accounts (Vardi 2011). In further developments, a motion has been filed against Full Tilt Poker alleging that the company operated a "global Ponzi scheme" using poker players' money to pay distributions totalling more than US$440 million to its board members and other owners and Alderney has revoked the sites license ('Alderney revokes Full Tilt' 2011; 'DoJ brings more charges' 2011). These examples demonstrate some of the potential risks associated with online gambling that players should be mindful of.

Unscrupulous operators can create online gambling sites for the purpose of defrauding and cheating customers. Typical examples include fraudulent "lottery scams", where an unlicensed illegal operator contacts individuals, typically via email, asking them to pay an amount of money as a handling fee or give personal information, including bank details, before a prize can be paid (European Commission 2011a). Such scams may attempt to replicate details of legitimate sites or gaming authorities. McMullen and Rege (2010) describe the case of MaxLotto, licensed in the Dominican Republic in 200; it advertised that 10% of its worldwide $100 million lottery revenues would be donated to charities. By 2002, however, MaxLotto had disappeared with all customer's money, no prizes paid out and no donations received. Phishing scams are also commonly aimed at the online gambling industry and players. For example, emails can promise individuals non-existent chip credits in order to gather genuine account credentials or identity and banking details through cloned site login screens (Winder 2011). Emails may also offer malware-infected software that claims to allow poker players to view opponent's hands or manipulate odds on a sports book. Further examples include emails informing individuals of lottery wins that include instructions to deposit funds for service charges into bank accounts in order to receive the jackpots (McMullen and Rege 2010).

Customer Protection

Further efforts by policy makers and operators are needed to educate individuals about the potential risks associated with online gambling. Jurisdictions that prohibit all or some Internet gambling sites should implement public education and awareness campaigns to inform individuals of the risks of playing on unregulated sites. This is particularly important for jurisdictions that encourage residents to use certain licensed sites, which abide by regulation and typically offer greater customer protection. Efforts undertaken to ensure that regulated sites offer strong customer protection measures may have minimal impact if unregulated and dubious sites are easily accessible and attractive to customers. Encouraging online gambling only on regulated sites and warnings about risks associated with unregulated sites should reduce the appeal of offshore sites for some players.

To ensure that an online gambling site is operated in an appropriate manner to uphold customer protection standards, a license should be provided by a stringent regulatory body. Most reputable jurisdictions have a common core of player protection strategies. Some jurisdictions, such as Alderney and the Isle of Man, are recognised for their high standards and requirements for operators to protect player funds and ensure that these are legally held in trust, rather than being used by the operators for other purposes. For example, PokerStars, regulated in the Isle of Man, was able to return player funds to individuals after the US indictments as all player accounts, including winnings, were held on the Isle of Man in a separate and segregated account, clearly designated as player funds and protected (Kimber 2011). As the industry matures, it is expected that consumers will increasingly recognise the importance of playing on regulated sites and demand high player protection standards from operators and governments. Online gambling operators should provide clear and easily accessible information about their regulatory and license requirements, including the jurisdiction in which they are licensed to customers and potential customers.

Site operators must also educate customers about potential risks, such as phishing threats, in order to protect themselves from loss of brand reputation and account hacking. Developing strong security teams and protocols is essential for ongoing success as an online gambling operator to develop and maintain customer trust and protect customers from potential abuse. This is likely to increase consumer trust and confidence as research indicates that Internet gamblers consider information presented on a website about the corporation, legal status and fairness of odds as the most important factor in judging the trustworthiness of a site (Shelat and Egger 2002). Seals and certificates of approval from third party organizations, such as eCOGRA, may also increase online vendor trust and favourable consumer perceptions regarding privacy policies, although only if customers are educated about the third party (Gainsbury et al. unpublished manuscript).

Unfair Player Practices

Unfair practices rest not only with the gaming operator but may also be found among the players themselves. The general lack of regulation of the online gambling industry, anonymity offered to players, and complications relating to international jurisdictions make online gambling sites vulnerable to player fraud and cheating. The AGA (2006) survey revealed that 46% of online gamblers believe that players have found a way to cheat the sites. With the increasing use of the Internet for commercial transactions, online purchases and online skill games, criminal theft and fraud including identity theft or the theft of virtual assets that can be readily sold remain significant concerns (Chen 2005).

Fraudulent online player gambling player behaviours include:

- Signing up for multiple casino accounts using different identities to claim a bonus multiple times;
- Disputing charges and failing to pay sites;
- Use of another person's credit card;
- Manipulation of gaming software or online sites – there have been several reports of hackers successfully manipulating online sites to pay winnings or cheat, such as changing odds of winning or allowing players to see their opponents hands (McMullen and Rege 2010; RSeconsulting 2006; Reuters 2001);
- Stealing virtual chips from player accounts or generating fake virtual chips (Winder 2011);
- Player collusion, where several online poker players at the same table are actually in the same physical location;
- Use of computer programs to facilitate optimal play against other players (e.g., poker bots). Individuals can create algorithms and software programs designed to monitor poker tables, memorise opponent's game styles and betting patterns, calculate the pot and hand odds of winning in an effort to play an optimal poker game (Brunker 2011; McMullen and Rege 2010);
- Use of laptops and mobile phones to place bets at sporting events (taking advantage of the several seconds delay between the time a point is scored on the court and the time the results takes effect on websites);
- Extortion of online sites by threatening to disrupt the site's online activity during major periods of business, in particular prior to major sporting events (McMullen and Rege 2010; RSeconsulting 2006; Williams and Wood 2007). Hundreds of gambling sites were subjected to denial of service attacks, and cyber-extortionists inflicted over $70 million in reported overall damages to British bookmakers alone in 2004 (McMullan and Rege 2010).

Criminal Transfers of Funds

Law enforcement officials are reportedly significantly concerned with the potential for Internet gambling to be a vehicle used by individuals and the sites themselves for laundering criminal proceeds and other forms of financial crime, including tax evasion (United States General Accounting Office 2002). The two main types of money laundering activity are complex transnational operations, designed to hide the criminal origins of large scale crimes to make the people and property involved appear legitimate, and any activity that conceals, disguises or disposes of the proceeds of any crime (European Commission 2011a). According to the US Government Audit Offices report to Congress, money laundering could be conducted through either legitimate or complicit sites that are knowingly working with criminals. Legitimate Internet gambling sites provide an opportunity to transfer high volumes of money in and out of accounts, with few wagers to mingle legitimate money with illicit funds, which would then be withdrawn through a different account under a false name. Individuals may not even have to place a wager, but could use online gambling accounts to store illicit funds before transferring them to an offshore account. In peer-to-peer online wagering, account holders can deliberately lose money to each other, paying just the house rake, and keeping potentially large sums of money that can then be claimed as gambling winnings.

The extent of such criminal activity is unknown but the Federal Bureau of Investigation has actively been involved in multiple cases and maintains a separate unit for this type of investigation. Reports from the multinational Financial Action Task Force (FATF) suggest that there is ample evidence of using Internet gambling to launder illicit funds (FATF 2001; United States Attorney 2008; US General Accounting Office 2002). Several cases have been reported of illegal money laundering and loan-sharking enterprises using online gambling sites (McMullen and Rege 2010). These include a case in which 40,000 fake accounts were created on a sports betting site used to launder criminal proceeds to offshore banks. In an example from New Zealand, a man has plead guilty to cheating investors out of nearly NZ$900,000 in a money-laundering and online sports betting scheme (Ihaka 2011). At least 200 small business are believed to have been invited to make deposits into a trading account, which they were told would be invested in a legitimate online Australian sports betting agency, International All Sports. However, after deposits were made the New Zealand-based was not able to be contacted. It is likely that similar schemes have occurred internationally.

Other Criminal Activity

Other crimes that may be linked to Internet gambling include the provision of gambling services by illegal operators, including criminal organisations and individuals, non-authorised Internet games offered by a licensed operator, and tax evasion

(European Commission 2011a). In 2011, a number of online gambling sites in the US were indicted and charged with bank fraud, money laundering and illegal gambling offenses (Ryan 2011). The Justice Department has filed a civil complaint for money laundering that seeks US$3 billion being held by the companies. According to a federal indictment, the owners of the companies sought ways to get around restrictions placed on US banks that prohibited them from handling financial transactions connected to online gambling. Some sites allegedly paid some banks a fee, others masked the transaction descriptions and arranged for money received from US gamblers to be disguised as payments to non-existent online merchants, such as flower delivery shops and pet supply stores. As mentioned above, Full Tilt Poker has been accused of operating a global Ponzi scheme using poker players' money to pay distributions totalling more than US$440 million to its board members and other owners ('DoJ brings more charges' 2011).

Fraud Detection and Anti-Money Laundering Strategies

Internet gambling sites have begun taking more precautions regarding licensing and registration measures and developed better internal security measures in an attempt to reduce the impact of criminal networks and malicious individuals. As Internet gambling sites typically require account holders to verify their identity and track customer behaviour, this electronic transaction record may take some steps towards reducing money laundering, at least on legitimate sites. The European Gaming and Betting Association, the Remote Gambling Association and the UK Gambling Commission have codes of conduct and documented policies and procedures to lower the risk of money laundering and criminal activities (Mangion 2010). Similarly, Australian gambling operators are required to report transactions over $10,000, international funds transfers, and suspicious transactions, such as cash transactions which fall just below the reporting limits (RSeConsulting 2006).

Many Internet gambling operators have sizeable security and fraud-detection departments. Operational practices to fight against money laundering include:

- Customer due diligence ensures that only registered players holding an account with the operator are allowed to play and information must be obtained to ensure that the player is the over the legal age limit to gamble, verify their identity, place of residence, a valid email address and valid form of payment, such as bank or credit card details. All identification details must be verified and checked, against third-party information where possible.
- Operators may monitor and take actions against customers that make substantial initial deposits, do not immediately place bets, or make withdrawals without placing any bets.
- Close screening and scrutiny of employees is also important to reduce potential threats from within an organisation. Staff should also undergo specific training concerning fraud and money laundering.

- Payment controls ensure that players always receive withdrawals by the same means in which the money was originally deposited and players cannot make direct payments to other customers.
- Operational controls including age verification lists and watch lists, such as those used by banks to identify terrorists.
- Operators keep records of all transactions, in compliance with data protection rules, in order to be able to identify suspicious activities, including irregular betting patterns.
- Stricter due diligence requirements may be required for products that have high limits on stakes.
- Operators must submit suspicious activity reports to the appropriate authorities.

The Study on Online Gambling commissioned by the European Parliament reported that there is no evidence to suggest that the online gambling industry is any more susceptible to problems of fraud and money laundering than other industries such as e-banking (European Parliament 2008). However, this applies to highly regulated sites such as those that are closely controlled in Europe. A particular problem with the enforcement of anti-money laundering regulations is that online gambling website frequently offer a variety of other (non-gambling services) and the operator may be licensed in more than one jurisdiction. A workshop held by the European Commission (2011c) concluded that cooperation between jurisdictions, operators and regulators as well as police and banks and that voluntary sharing of information was highly important. This should include investigations into offshore jurisdictions and joint efforts to fight illegal online gambling.

One significant difficulty in combating cybercrime is that regulations are largely unclear and can be difficult to enforce in an international market. Laws are imprecise on whether crimes should be prosecuted in the country where criminal networks are based, or in the jurisdiction where the crimes happened (McMullan and Rege 2010). Many police forces do not have the reach and resources or expertise to investigate crimes that were committed from offshore jurisdictions.

Players can also take steps to protect themselves from potential fraud and deception. In a document published by the UK Gambling Commission (2008), 'What to look out for when gambling online', they recommend that players should consider when selecting an Internet gambling site: (a) is the operator licensed by a regulator, (b) where are the different gambling products regulated (many Internet gambling companies are regulated in more than one jurisdiction, as such certain games may be regulated in different jurisdictions), (c) look for details about the company (e.g., where they are licensed and how you can contact them), (d) check forums where you can acquire information about the site, (e) are the company's terms and conditions easily available and clearly explained, (f) determine if your money is refunded if the company becomes insolvent, (g) does the company ensure your personal details are safe, (h) are there measures in place to help you gamble responsibly, (i) check to ensure that the rules of the game are clearly explained, and (j) does the software and game meet minimal technical requirements established by the regulator and does it include independent testing. The Gambling Commission clearly suggests that consumers be aware and that caution is warranted before engaging in online gambling.

Chapter 6
Vulnerable Populations

Abstract Internet gambling lacks the gate-keeping systems of land-based gambling venues that protect vulnerable individuals. Internet gambling poses particular risks to two specific vulnerable populations; youth and problem gamblers. Adolescents and young adults are familiar with Internet technology and appear to be gambling online at higher rates than the general adult population. This is particularly concerning as gambling at an early age is associated with gambling problems and engagement with gambling at a young age may lead to increased involvement during adulthood. Internet gambling has been associated with problem gambling as higher rates of problem gamblers have been found in samples of Internet gamblers. It is likely that problem gamblers use this mode of gambling when other forms are not available and therefore, Internet gambling acts to maintain and exacerbate existing problems. However, Internet gambling is also likely to create problems for individuals who would not gamble on other means and cause substantial difficulties. This chapter outlines the specific risks posed by online gambling to adolescents and young adults and the use of online gambling amongst these populations. The impact of advertising and marketing on youth is also explored, including measures that should be enacted to protect this group. The impact of Internet gambling on problem gambling is also explored. Research findings are critically analyzed as well as factors that appear to be associated with Internet gambling problems.

Keywords Internet gambling • Online gaming • Youth • Adolescents • Young adults • Students • Problem Gambling • Risk factors • Self exclusion • Advertising

There are many groups of individuals that may be particularly vulnerable to Internet gambling-related harms. Potentially vulnerable groups of people include adolescents, young adults and inexperienced gamblers, problem gamblers, drug and alcohol users and those with previous addiction problems, the learning impaired, and those with easy access to gambling or links with events on which bets are placed

S. Gainsbury, *Internet Gambling: Current Research Findings and Implications*,
SpringerBriefs in Behavioral Medicine 1, DOI 10.1007/978-1-4614-3390-3_6,
© Springer Science+Business Media, LLC 2012

(European Commission 2011a). Some of these groups would be prevented from gambling in land-based venues by responsible gambling policies (Griffiths 2003). As the online gambling industry matures, efforts are increasingly being made by many responsible operators to take advantage of customer identification procedures to detect individuals that may be at risk of harm and implement measures to protect these individuals.

Nonetheless, concerns have been raised that some less scrupulous Internet gambling operators may unfairly target vulnerable populations with misleading advertisements and other practices, such as not verifying customer age, address, and identity and not providing responsible gambling tools. For example, an Internet advertising campaign for an online gambling site was removed from circulation in the UK by the Advertising Standards Authority (Gaming Zion 2011). The most problematic advertisement featured an image of a woman holding a baby. The text read: "*I am a single mom & I live on family benefits, I played and won £46,799 and it is incredible for me. I was very stressed for my son's future and I couldn't sleep, now that I won I know that I can help my son build a better future.*" This advertisement was deemed to exploit vulnerable people by claiming to offer a solution to debt. The advertisements were viewed more than a billion times before they were pulled, clearly demonstrating the importance of vigilance by regulators to monitor marketing practices and take steps to protect vulnerable groups as much as possible from the potential harms of online gambling.

Limited customer information is gathered to create online betting accounts and it can be argued that it is difficult for online operators to identify all customers that may be at-risk without a centralised database of vulnerable individuals. It is also difficult for an online gambling operator to verify whether the individual placing bets is actually the account holder, whether they are of the legal age to gamble, or whether they are gambling whilst intoxicated. Nonetheless, efforts should be made by regulators, operators, and researchers to understand how vulnerable populations may be impacted by Internet gambling and what measure may protect them from harm.

Adolescents and Young Adults

Adolescents who would typically be prevented from gambling in land-based venues appear to be engaging in Internet gambling. Research indicates that underage youth are gambling online at higher rates than adults. Studies in the US, UK, Canada, Sweden, and Australia report that 4–19% of adolescents and 3–33% of young adults have gambled online (Delfabbro et al. 2005; Jackson et al. 2008; McBride and Derevensky 2009; MORI/International Gaming Research Unit 2006; Petry and Weinstock 2007; Swedish National Institute of Public Health 2011; Wood et al. 2007). For example, studies reported that 6% of high school students in New York State gambled online in the past year (Rainone and Gallati 2007) and 9% of Canadian high-school students reporting having gambled for money on the Internet; an increase from 3.6% in 2005, with over half of those surveyed also reporting playing on 'practice' sites (Derevensky 2009; MacKay 2005; McBride 2006). A 2006 study in Nova Scotia, Canada reported that 12% of 10–20 year olds, 19% of 15–17 year olds, and 15% of 18 year olds indicated they had gambled online (Meerkamper 2006). Although these figures include individuals who played without money, these are significantly higher rates of online gambling than found among adults. The 2007 adult gambling prevalence survey reported that only 1.6% of Nova Scotian adults had ever gambled on non-regulated Internet sites, and 2.1% had gambled on ALC's online gambling site (Focal Research Consultants 2008).

In a 2003–2004 study involving more than 900 Australian secondary school students, 6.1% of students had gambled on the Internet in the past year (Delfabbro et al. 2005). In another Australian study with 2,766 eighth-grade students (mean age 14 years), 4% had gambled online in the past year, with males significantly more likely to do so (Jackson et al. 2008). Similar findings have been reported in the UK In a study with over 8,000, 12–15 year olds, 8% of the youth reported playing the National lottery online, despite the minimum legal age to play being 16, with boys more likely to report online gambling than girls (10% and 6% respectively) (MORI/ International Gaming Research Unit 2006). Young people identified as problem gamblers were more likely than social gamblers to have played the lottery game on the Internet (37% versus 9%). Of those youth who played the National Lottery online, 29% reported also playing free games on the Internet, 18% reported the system let them register, 16% played with their parents, 10% used their parent's account with permission, while 7% played without their parent's permission. These results indicate that school-aged children and adolescents are gambling online on both free-play and money sites through a variety of methods, suggesting that current age verification measures are not sufficiently effective in preventing underage play.

Young adults are also gambling online; in a study of Internet gambling among 1,356 US university undergraduates, 23% reported having gambled on the Internet, with 6.3% reported doing so weekly (Petry and Weinstock 2007). Increased frequency of Internet was associated with problem gambling; almost two-thirds (61.6%) of regular Internet gamblers were pathological gamblers, compared with 23.9% of infrequent Internet gamblers and 5.0% of non-Internet gamblers. Internet gamblers were more likely to be younger, male, and have poorer grades. Internet gambling frequency was found to be significantly associated with mental health issues after controlling for demographic and pathological gambling. Frequent Internet gamblers also wagered more often than other groups when all types of gambling were considered. On a positive note, more than half of the frequent Internet gamblers (61.2%) revealed that they would be interested in acquiring information about problem gambling and ways to reduce their gambling (in contrast to 38.4% of infrequent and 19.2% of youth who never gambled on the Internet).

Similarly, in a study of 465 students (aged 18–20 years) recruited from English speaking universities in Montreal, Canada, 8% reported having gambled for money on the Internet and 43% of students reported playing on practice sites during the past year (McBride and Derevensky 2009). The most popular reasons cited for Internet gambling were similar to those given by adults: for the competition (60%)

(especially true for card players), convenience (40%), 24-h accessibility (33%), privacy (33%), high speed of play (33%), good odds (33%), fair/reliable payouts (33%), bonus money (27%), graphics (20%), sex appeal (20%), and anonymity (20%) (McBride and Derevensky 2009). Among individuals identified as problem gamblers, 60% reported that the thrill and rush associated with Internet gambling centred upon competition and the competitiveness of the games, indicating that problem gamblers may be playing games with an element of skill involved, such as betting or poker. A UK study of college students found that a third of individuals played Internet poker at least twice a week and nearly one-fifth (18%) were identified as problem gamblers (Wood et al. 2007).

However, in contrast to results from samples recruited from school-based populations, a large international survey of gamblers found that only 0.4% of Internet gamblers were under the age of 18, a rate even lower than that observed among non-Internet gamblers (Wood and Williams 2011). The different methods of recruitment are likely to influence these results; however, it does question the age profile of Internet gamblers and the extent to which underage youth are gambling online. Similarly, despite research results such as those presented above, online gambling does not appear to be a significant concern for parents, teachers or treatment providers (Derevensky 2009). Since the introduction of laws requiring rigorous age verification for all sites licensed in the UK, the Children's Charities' Coalition on Internet Safety reports that no cases of children accessing Internet gambling sites have been raised (Carr 2011). These results may indicate that adults are unaware of youth online gambling or that there is a discrepancy between school-based studies and actual behaviour.

Increases in Internet gambling availability may increase youth participation. For example, studies in Iceland found that one fourth of adolescents surveyed in 2007–2008 had wagered money on the Internet compared to one fifth of adolescents surveyed in 2006 and only 2% in studies from 2003 to 2004 (Olason et al. 2011). This trend occurred whilst there was a downward trend in adolescent gambling on gaming machines, scratch tickets and lotto. These changes reportedly coincided with considerable increase in the access and quality of Internet connections available in Icelandic homes. In 2002, about 78% of Icelandic homes had access to the Internet but only 26% were connected with high speed connections. In 2006, the number of Internet connected homes had risen to 84% and 85% of connected homes had high speed Internet connections (Statistics Iceland 2006). In a sample of 1,887 adolescents recruited from Icelandic schools in 2007–2008, 24.3% reported wagering money on gambling websites and 4.1% did so at least weekly (Olason et al. 2011). Older adolescents (15–18 years) and boys were more likely to gamble online and online gamblers were more likely to also gamble on land-based games (95.1% vs. 42.1%). The most popular forms of Internet gambling were casino type games on non-Icelandic websites, Internet Lotto and sports pools on Icelandic websites. Consistent with other international findings, the prevalence of problem gambling amongst Internet gamblers (7.5%) was considerably higher than for the total sample (2.2%) or land-based only gamblers (1.1%). Further analyses revealed that adolescents who gambled online in addition to land-based gambling were most likely to be classified as problem (7.7%) or high-risk (10.6%) gamblers.

Given the experience of adolescents and young adults and their familiarity with computer use, the Internet in general and experience playing video games it should not be surprising that youth and young adults are engaging in Internet gambling as they are primed for this activity. Results from the Pew Internet and American Life Project found that in 2007–2008, 93% of teenagers between the ages of 12 and 17 reported using the Internet, an increase from 73% in 2001 (Pew Internet and American Life Project 2001, 2009). Similar access rates have been found worldwide with a survey of adolescents in 13 countries observing that 100% of 12–14 year olds have Internet access in the UK, followed by 98% in the Czech Republic, 96% in Macau, and 95% in Canada (Centre for the Digital Future 2008). Even in the countries with the least Internet access usage was still common with 70% of adolescents in Hungary and Singapore reporting regular Internet use.

Age restrictions on legal land-based gambling opportunities might make Internet gambling more attractive for youth, as age restrictions are easier to circumvent on online gambling sites and the possibility of anonymity is greater than in land-based activities (Derevensky and Gupta 2007; Griffiths and Barnes 2008). Although most online sites report prohibiting individuals younger than 18 from gambling, few sites have highly reliable measures to assess the age and identity of the individual actively gambling online at any one time. A study conducted in the UK found that a 16 year old was able to place bets online on 81% (30 out of 37) sites tested and a European survey reported 17% of visitors to online gambling sites were under the age of 18 (NCH 2004; 'Europeans take a gamble' 2002). Among a sample of online gamblers there was widespread belief that underage players are gambling online, and several participants reported noticing fellow gamblers soliciting help for their homework via chat boxes (Cotte and Latour 2009).

More recently improved efforts by online gambling sites to identify customers have reduced the ease with which an under aged person could open an account for gambling and withdraw winnings (European Commission 2011a). Many operators do make efforts to verify a customer's age and identity before they set up an account and place bets. For example, customers may be required to provide copies of identity documents (e.g., driver's licence, passport, etc.,) and payment details such as credit card and bank accounts can be verified. In Australia, Internet gambling providers are required to verify a person's ID within 90 days of the account being opened or must freeze the account and payments cannot be made to the player unless evidence of ID has been obtained. Although underage gamblers can technically open an account and make (and lose bets) within this 3 month period, the inability to withdraw any winnings is clearly stated in an attempt to discourage such behaviour. Consequently, should an underage person seek to gamble online (using an adult's credit card), they will not be able to activate their account until their name, address and date of birth has been verified. However, it is possible that an underage person may obtain the details of an adult's account or create an account on a site with fewer identification requirements. In the UK, third party groups can cross-check customer data with public data to confirm that the registered customer is the right person. This process takes place in real time and has achieved successful matching rates over 90%; this process is particularly successful in keeping children off gambling websites (EGBA 2011). It is not certain how various operators manage accounts created with pre-paid credit cards as these are generally not linked to an identified individual and can essentially be used to gamble online anonymously (Carr 2011).

The reasons adolescents are not permitted to gamble online are the same as for land-based forms of gambling and are similar to the reason gambling amongst young adults should be discouraged; the cognitive development, attitudes and perceptions amongst youth means that they are more likely to be engaged in risk-taking behaviours, they perceive themselves to be smarter and more invulnerable than the general population, and they are more easily impacted by the sensitive advertisements (Monaghan and Derevensky 2008).

Although there is some evidence to indicate that youth are gambling online, and may be doing so at potentially higher rates than other age cohorts, the impact of Internet gambling in this population is still unclear. Reports from gambling treatment centres in Australia and New Zealand suggest that there is an increase in numbers of youth seeking help for Internet gambling, although the total number of online Internet gamblers and young adults seeking help for gambling problems remains low ('Online gambling strife' 2011; Problem Gambling Foundation 2011; University of Sydney 2011). However, few youth seek treatment for gambling problems and gambling problems may not develop for several years as youth have fewer resources to spend (Derevensky and Gupta 2002). Therefore, it is possible that if Internet gambling continues to be popular amongst youth and the general population, treatment seeking for online gambling problems will increase in subsequent years. Adolescents and young adults who bet online may be more likely to be problem gamblers, have greater levels of impulsivity, poor academic outcomes, engage in delinquent activities, abuse alcohol and illicit drugs, experience psychological distress and take medication for depression and anxiety (MacKay 2005; Mihaylova and Kairouz 2010; Petry and Weinstock 2007). This suggests that all adolescents seen by health or mental health workers for non-gambling related issues should also be screened for potential Internet gambling involvement as an early detection and prevention measure.

Practice Sites

Practice sites provide an avenue for gambling operators to advertise, particularly in jurisdictions that prohibit advertising of gambling sites. Professional, high-profile gamblers are often paid to wear clothing that markets practice sites during televised poker tournaments and appeal to youth as an icon to emulate. Advertisements for "free sites" appear frequently on Internet sites as well as on television, magazines, billboards, and radio stations that value and target a youth audience (Monaghan et al. 2009). The use of practice/trial sites is also of considerable concern as these sites incorporate identical games to gambling sites, often encourage individuals to play online by providing free promotional material, have over-inflated pay-out rates, and are perceived to be a training ground for wagering with money (Monaghan et al. 2009). Simulated gambling on practice sites may build self-confidence and potentially increase one's illusion of control in determining gambling outcomes – motivating participation in their real money counterparts. Canadian research indicates that problem gamblers are more likely than at-risk and social gamblers to use free practice sites, and begin using these sites at a young age (less than ten) (Derevensky 2009). A survey conducted in the US found that 33% of youths aged 12–17 gamble online for free and Canadian studies reported that half of youth surveyed reported playing on free-money sites (Derevensky 2008; Kim 2008; MacKay 2005; McBride 2006).

Advertising Restrictions to Protect Youth

Research indicates that youth are highly influenced by gambling advertising (Lamont et al. 2011; Monaghan et al. 2009). Studies involving Canadian adolescents report that advertisements for gambling products increases the extent to which youth think about and want to try gambling as well as the likelihood of youth engaging in gambling (Derevensky et al. 2010; Felsher et al. 2004). Promotional products, sexualised images, and celebrity endorsements appear to be highly appealing to youth (Monaghan et al. 2009) and these techniques may encourage adolescents and young adults to engage in gambling, particularly online gambling due to its accessibility.

Although adolescents possess the cognitive abilities to comprehend and evaluate advertising, at this developmental stage they are more persuaded by the emotive content of commercials that play into their concerns regarding appearance, self-identity, belonging, and sexuality (Story and French 2004). Evidence of adolescents' cognitive processing of advertisements is shown in research findings suggesting that although many adolescents report being aware that messages promoted are unrealistic, they are still heavily influenced by them (Derevensky et al. 2007). Korn (2005) reported the messages adolescents perceived from marketing campaigns are that gambling is enjoyable and entertaining, it is easy to win, anyone can win, it is rewarding and life-changing, and it benefits society. The motivations reported as leading youth to gamble – fun and excitement, possible financial gain, lifestyle or status attainment, and a way to facilitate socialising – directly paralleled the messages obtained from advertisements.

Over the recent years online gambling operators have become a significant corporate sponsor of sports teams and events (Lamont et al. 2011). For example, in 2009 14 of the 16 teams in one of the major Australian professional rugby competitions had sponsorship arrangements with gambling operators, including online gambling operators, many of which wear the company logos on their jerseys (Lamont et al. 2011). Concerns are increasingly being voiced by communities and other stakeholder groups including sporting organisations and politicians over the increasing promotion of online gambling during sporting broadcasts and the potential negative influence that this may have. For example, the Crawford Report

(Independent Sports Panel 2009), noted concerns within the Australian community about 'mixed messages' sent by governments about the benefits of a healthy, active lifestyle, while allowing gambling operators to sponsor sport.

Some regulations have been enacted to limit the advertisement of gambling products. For example, in the UK and Australia, general advertising of gambling products is banned in multiple forms of media, and casinos and bookmakers have been banned from advertising on television before 9 p.m. (Office of Public Sector Information 2005; Totalizator Regulation 2005). Although these restrictions do not apply to bingo, lottery and sports betting during televised events, which may suggest to youth that these activities are perceived as more acceptable. In the UK and Australia, child-size replica sports jerseys for some sports are not permitted to include logos of online gambling operators (Office of Public Sector Information 2005; Victorian Commission for Gambling Regulation 2011). In August 2011, the Melbourne Cricket Ground (MCG) Trust banned the promotion of live odds gambling during Australian Football League matches at the MCG next season after the current contract has expired (Victorian Commission for Gambling Regulation 2011). This is now consistent with Cricket Australia and the National Rugby League, which do not allow the promotion of live odds and is based on increasing concerns at the rapid increase in the promotion of gambling during matches, especially live betting odds. However, given the high number of sponsorship deals internationally between sporting teams and events and online gambling operators, youth are still faced with high levels of exposure to promotions of this form of gambling. For example, one sports stadium in Sydney was renamed Centrebet Stadium, following a sponsorship deal with the prominent online bookmaker and many sporting codes display betting odds prominently on their websites.

The UK has also been quite active in banning advertisements that are misleading about the chances of winning or appeal to children. For example, a gambling advertisement by Paddy Power was banned on grounds that it was irresponsible in claiming that online betting would improve sexual prowess and self-esteem and that it featured slapstick, juvenile humour that was likely to appeal to children (Reuters 2008). The advertisement was published in the Times and featured a dwarf in a limousine flanked by two beautiful women, smoking a cigar and holding a champagne glass with the tagline "Who says you can't make money being short?" A campaign by InterCasino featuring dwarves undertaking "Jackass-style" stunts was also banned for appealing to children or young people (Reuters 2008). Despite the advertisements being banned, they are typically widely viewed, and some operators, such as Paddy Power appear to deliberately create controversial advertisements and perhaps benefit from the publicity gained from regulator scrutiny. Many advertising campaigns for online gambling sites feature celebrities that are likely to be appealing to adolescents and young adults such as those featuring Brooke Burke (America's best-selling calendar model and hostess of popular E!'s Wild on…), and Nikki Cox (star of the popular television show Las Vegas). Young people may also aspire to the numerous celebrities and professional poker players featured in television shows, including televised poker tournaments and games.

The impacts of advertisements for online gambling include that this activity is increasingly normalised and seen as acceptable by children, adolescents and young adults, which may increase the likelihood that they will engage in online gambling. In an effort to reduce the appeal of online gambling to under aged minors restrictions can be placed on advertising and marketing efforts by online gambling operators (Monaghan et al. 2009). Examples of appropriate advertising and promotion rules include:

- Gambling advertisements should not be directed to those aged below the national age limit for gambling.
- Gambling advertisements should not be broadcast or communicated during programmes aimed towards young people on mainstream channels, or for certain periods of time before such programs.
- People depicted in gambling advertisements must appear well above the national age limit for gambling.
- Gambling advertisements should not be appealing to children or young persons, e.g., by being associated with youth culture.
- Gambling advertisements should not feature celebrities popular amongst youth.
- Gambling advertisements should not be displayed close to areas which children frequent, potentially including prominent advertising in sports stadiums.
- Free-play or practice sites should be subjected to the same advertising restrictions as gambling sites.
- Advertisements for gambling products must contain accurate information regarding the chances of winning and a visible warning statement that highlights the potential risks associated with excessive gambling.

Problem Gamblers

Politicians, advocates and researchers have expressed concerns about the potential public health impact of Internet gambling (European Commission 2011a; Gainsbury 2010; Griffiths 2001, 2003; LaBrie et al. 2007; Productivity Commission 2010). Problematic behaviour on the Internet is not unique to gambling. Similar to problem gamblers, excessive Internet users have reported time disorientation and unsuccessful attempts to reduce their Internet use despite the significant problems it was causing (Young 1998a, b). Furthermore, excessive Internet use has been associated with subjective distress, considerable social, vocational and/or financial impairment, as well as substantial psychiatric comorbidity (Shapira et al. 2001). This suggests that certain features of the Internet may interact with gambling to produce negative consequences for players (Monaghan 2009b).

Examples of the characteristics of Internet gambling that are of greatest concern due to their potential propensity to facilitate problem gambling are similar to the factors that are cited as benefits to the majority of customers. These include:

- Convenience and accessibility – unlimited access to gambling opportunities from almost any location, no restrictions on duration of play, allowing short and long sessions (Wood and Williams 2007; Wood, Williams et al. 2007)

- Electronic payment – ability to purchase gambling through credit cards and online banking systems, electronic payment may have a lower 'psychological value' than cash (Griffiths 2003)
- Choice – easy access to an increasing number of games and gambling products, many of which may be unavailable in local jurisdiction, with a wide range of player protection strategies appeal of technology, multi-lingual option and play against gamblers from around the world, ability to play multiple games simultaneously (Griffiths and Wood 2000; Monaghan 2009b)
- Cost – Low outlays to access gambling, ability to play for low stakes, competitive odds, bonuses and free credits (McCormack and Griffiths 2011; Wood, Williams et al. 2007)
- Environment – anonymity of use, absence of screening that occurs in some venues for intoxication, age, or exclusion, ability to play in comfortable environment, may reduce social stigma and allow novices to try new games (Cotte and Latour 2009; Griffiths and Barnes 2008; Lloyd et al. 2010; McCormack and Griffiths 2011 ; Wood, Williams et al. 2007)
- The immersive nature of the Internet may result in dissociation and players losing track of time and money spent, which may facilitate the emergence of a gambling problem (Griffiths 2003; Griffiths and Parke 2002; Monaghan 2009b).
- Interaction – opportunity to choose level of interaction preferred, from high to low, increased ability to play against a wider range of players, high-speed game options, prevalence of advertising and inducement from operators (Corney and Davis 2010; Cotte and Latour 2009; Wood and Griffiths 2008)

As with offline gambling, some game types may be associated with a greater propensity to result in negative consequences. It has been argued that games that are continuous, with short intervals between bet placement and determination of outcome and utilize variable ratio schedules of reinforcement, such as casino games, slots, or keno are more likely to lead to gambling problems than games such as poker, racing and sports wagering and traditional lottery draws, which occur more slowly with clearly defined outcomes (Breen and Zimmerman 2002; Turner 2008). Highly volatile games, such as slots, lotteries and bingo, have frequent small prizes and infrequent large wins and may encourage greater variation in bet sizes leading to increased losses and subsequent gambling problems (Holtgrave 2009; Turner 2008). Continuous and rapid games are also argued to foster irrational and superstitious beliefs, erroneous concepts of probability, randomness and mutual independence that contribute to illusions of control and the maintenance of problem gambling (Ladouceur et al. 2001). These types of products may produce dissociative states, including losing track of time, going into a trance-like state, feeling like a different person, experience blackouts, and feeling 'outside' oneself (Powell et al. 1996) during play. The technological and product sophistication of Internet gambling options means that many traditionally slower games may now be played at higher speeds and bets placed more quickly, for example, live action and micro betting on in-play outcomes, ability to bet on events around the world, instant lottery draws and scratch tickets, and playing multiple poker tables, simultaneously. This may widen the types of gambling associated with problems and create difficulties for people that gambled to a lesser extent on offline forms.

Recent increases in media attention, has heightened public interest in and concern about online gambling. In a series of interviews with 29 gamblers (Internet and land-based) and 11 non-gamblers, a clear trend emerged in responses indicating a perception that Internet gambling is more addictive and potentially dangerous for vulnerable people, and will ultimately exacerbate gambling problems in society (McCormack and Griffiths 2010). The recruitment source of these participants is not described, but it is presumed that they were based in the UK, due to the location of the study's authors. However, in contrast, an Australian public opinion poll found that only 1% of participants regarded 'casino type games on the Internet for money' to be most related to gambling problems and only 6% of participants listed it as the second most common cause of gambling problems (Australian National Institute for Public Policy 2011). This indicates that public perception of Internet-related gambling problems may still lag behind concerns about more popular forms traditionally associated with harm, such as electronic gaming machines.

Prevalence of Internet Gambling Problems

The concern about Internet gambling is largely based on various international research studies that have found relatively high rates of problem gambling among samples of Internet gamblers as compared to the general population and in some instances, non-Internet gamblers. Some of these results are summarised in Table 6.1.

As can be seen from Table 6.1, the levels of problem gambling amongst Internet gamblers is not fixed, but there is some evidence that those who have gambled online are more likely to have gambling problems than land-based gamblers. When interpreting data across studies, it is important to note that the varied methodology and measures used mean that the results are not always easily comparable. Some studies did not include control or comparison groups, or recruited particularly involved Internet gamblers and the samples may not be representative of the wider population of Internet gamblers. It is also important to consider that, although Internet gamblers appear to be more likely to have gambling problems when compared to the general adult population or a sample of non-gamblers, when compared to other groups of regular gamblers, this difference may not be significant. For example, in an Australian study of gamblers, 9.6% of Internet gamblers appeared to have gambling problems, which is greater than the level of problems reported by the small sample of land-based gamblers. However, Internet gamblers appeared to have lower problem gambling rates than the level of gambling problems reported by regular gamblers (15.4%) in the general population (Allen Consulting Group 2003). Furthermore, as demonstrated above, Internet gamblers have a tendency to gamble on a wide range of activities, rather than

Table 6.1 Prevalence of problem gambling in Internet gambling samples

Sample	Problem gambling prevalence amongst Internet gamblers (%)	Comparative problem gambling prevalence rate	Measure	Reference
7,921 International gamblers	3.8	1.7% land-based gamblers	PGSI 8+	Wood and Williams (2011)
473 university student Internet gamblers, UK	5.5	None	SOGS 5+	Griffiths and Barnes (2008)
9,003 adults, UK	3.8	0.1% non-Internet gamblers (including land-based gamblers and non-gamblers)	DSM-IV criteria 5+	Griffiths et al. (2009a)
1,920 Internet gamblers	20.1	None	PGSI 8+	Wood and Williams (2007)
2,002 Swedish Internet poker players	8			Jonsson (2008)
179 online poker players	9	None	PGSI 8+	Hopley and Nicki (2010)
563 online gamblers	11	None	DSM-IV criteria 5+	McBride and Derevensky (2009)
1,537 Icelandic youth	7.7	1.1% land-based gamblers	DSM-IV-MR-J 4+	Olason et al. (2011)
4,636 Norweigans 15 years+	13.6			Rogge and Ukkelberg (2010)
2,081 Australians	9.6	2.3% land-based gamblers	SOGS 5+	Allen Consulting Group (2003)
389 dental clinic patients	64.5	11.1% land-based gamblers	SOGS 5+	Ladd and Petry (2002)

being purely online gamblers. This makes it difficult to determine the form and mode of gambling that makes the most significant contribution to their problems reported.

The causality of problems associated with online gambling has yet to be determined, with preliminary results indicating that there is a bi-directional effect; that is, Internet gambling may cause problems for some that have no previously experienced problems, and it may also exacerbate problems for those that have existing difficulties. This is a highly important area for future research as it has implications for Internet gambling policies as well as prevention, public education, and responsible gambling strategies to be implemented.

The trend toward legalization and concomitant increased availability, promotion and widespread market penetration of new forms of gambling have also been anticipated to lead to a resurgent incidence of problem gambling (Abbott et al. 2004; Toneatto and Ladouceur 2003; Welte et al. 2009). There have been anecdotal reports of increases in the number of treatment-seeking gamblers citing Internet gambling as the most problematic forms. Data from the Swedish national gambling helpline indicates that in 2010, 44% of callers reported Internet gambling as their main problem, compared to 39% for electronic gaming machines (Svensson and Romild 2011). Others have argued that gamblers adapt to gambling opportunities over time and rates of problem gambling may reduce in response to responsible gambling strategies and consumer protection policies (LaPlante and Shaffer 2007; Shaffer and Martin 2011). It is also possible that as participation in Internet gambling increases that the general public's participation may to some extent dilute the proportion of Internet gamblers that are problem gamblers (Allen Consulting Group 2003). Despite widely cited concerns over the potential for Internet gambling to dramatically increase the number of people experiencing gambling problems, there is little evidence to indicate that the prevalence of problem gambling has increased worldwide, or in countries that have liberalised access to online gambling. A report based on one workshop held by the European Commission to discuss Internet gambling says that access to online gambling products "does not appear to have given rise to problem development or addiction at a higher rate than in the offline environment" (European Commission 2011b).

Nonetheless, given the substantial annual social cost associated with problem gambling, estimated to approximate AUD$4.7 billion annually in Australia (Productivity Commission 2010), coupled with the personal and familial distress any activity that contributes to gambling problems should be addressed. The fluctuation of prevalence rates is, from a public health perspective, irrelevant since the absolute number of individuals requiring treatment is substantial and represents (and is predicted to remain) a major health and social burden (Monaghan and Blaszczynski 2010b). The European Commission's workshop on prevention of Internet gambling problems suggested that regulated online gambling "provides good opportunities for close monitoring of individual gambling behaviour and early detection of problem development" and that measure should be taken by operators and regulators to reduce potential harms (European Commission 2011b).

Factors Associated with Internet Gambling Problems

In a survey of 1,920 Internet gamblers, 42.7% of participants were classified as at-moderate-risk or probably problem gamblers (Wood and Williams 2007). Analysis of game preference found that certain forms of games were favoured by problem gamblers including Baccarat, Pai Gow Poker, Caribbean Poker, Craps, and Keno, although sport betting, Blackjack and Roulette were also played by a large proportion of problem gamblers. These games include a mixture of skill and chance-based games, although all can be played at high levels of intensity with frequent bets possible. Interestingly, a preference for non-Internet gambling was identified among the variables that reliably predicted problem gambling status amongst Internet gamblers. This may support the view that problem gamblers naturally gravitate to online gambling as simply one more gambling opportunity rather the Internet games being a cause of problems.

A study of 1,015 treatment-seeking gamblers, including 53 gamblers that played online, was conducted in a public hospital in Barcelona (Jiménez-Murcia et al. 2011). The majority (51%) of the online problem gamblers were engaged in sports betting, 41% played poker or card games and 32% played online casino games. The online problem gamblers had higher education levels and sociodemographic status as well as higher maximum amounts and higher average amounts spent gambling and higher gambling debts as compared to non-online problem gamblers. However, no significant differences were found in any of the psychopathology or personality traits measured or other gambling or sociodemographic variables. This study did not examine causality, and it is possible that Internet gamblers have greater education and socio-economic levels as these is generally related to Internet gambling use. However, as the online problem gamblers did not also play land-based games, it does provide some insight in the differences between online and non-online cohorts of problem gamblers. The results indicate that online problem gamblers are not substantially different to non-online problem gamblers, suggesting that similar treatment programs may be effective for both groups.

In a small study with 25 female Internet gamblers in the UK, of the 16 problem gamblers, 6 participants stated that had gambling problems prior to gambling online, 10 did not appear to have problems prior to Internet gambling and 2 had very little gambling experience prior to starting online gambling (Corney and Davis 2010). Participants reported that the factors that increased their problems included not perceiving online expenditure as "real" money, losing track of expenditure and playing multiple online games, which also increased expenditure. The Internet gamblers indicated that gambling problems developed relatively quickly after commencing online play, within 2–4 months, and were primarily driven by a desire to escape and seek relief from their problems and also by experiencing early and big wins, that encouraged continued play.

A prevalence study in Norway found that problem gamblers were overrepresented among Internet gamblers including those who play poker online at least weekly (13.6% vs. 2% of the population), gamblers on foreign sports sites (10.4% vs. 0%)

and Internet casino games (6.1%) (Rogge and Ukkelberg 2010). Those at risk for gambling problems were four times more likely to gambling online compared to the non-risk group (29.9% vs. 7.3%) and to gambled using mobile phones (3.0% vs. 0.7%). Problem gamblers reported spending significantly more time and money gambling online each week than non-problem gamblers and were more likely to be experiencing negative consequences of online gambling.

In a large International sample of gamblers recruited from a popular online gambling portal, 16.4% of Internet gamblers were either at moderate risk or possible problem gamblers, compared to a rate of 5.7% among non-Internet gamblers (Wood and Williams 2011). Only 39.9% of Internet gamblers were classified as non-problem gamblers, which is less than half the rate of 82.1% observed among their non-Internet gambling counterparts. In this study, approximately half the Internet problem gamblers reported that there was a specific type of gambling that contributed to their problems, with gaming machines (23.8%), poker (21.7%) and Internet gambling (11.3%) being the most commonly reported. This survey provided some support for the claim that people vulnerable to developing gambling problems may be more likely to gamble online, and that reported problems relate to land-based forms. Internet gamblers reported higher rates of tobacco, alcohol and drug use and had higher rates of substance and other addictions than non-Internet gamblers (Wood and Williams 2010). Participants demonstrated some awareness of the potential risks of online gambling with 19% reporting that it was easier to spend more money online compared to offline, 16% reporting it was 'too convenient' and 12% stating that it was more addictive. A small proportion of Internet gamblers reported that the use of electronic money tended to increase their spending (10%) and that Internet gambling disrupted their sleep (11%) and eating (4%).

Amalgamating results across various studies, several variables appear to increase the likelihood of an Internet gambler being classified as a problem gambler. These include:

- Being male (Wood and Williams 2007)
- Gambling on a greater number of gambling formats (Wardle et al. 2011a; Wood and Williams 2010)
- Higher gambling expenditure (McBride and Derevensky 2009; Wood and Williams 2010)
- Longer gambling sessions (Hopley and Nicki 2010; McBride and Derevensky 2009; Wood and Williams 2007)
- More frequent gambling sessions (Hopley and Nicki 2010)
- Gambling alone (McBride and Derevensky 2009)
- Spending over allocated time and budget
- Having a greater number of gambling-related irrational beliefs
- Having co-morbid mental health problems (Wood and Williams 2010)
- Having a family history of problem gambling (Wood and Williams 2010)
- Being single (Wood and Williams 2010)
- Lower household income (Wood and Williams 2010)

- Use alcohol or drugs when gambling online (McBride and Derevensky 2009)
- Having a history of addiction (Wood and Williams 2010)
- Experiencing dissociation, boredom proneness, impulsivity (Hopley and Nicki 2010)
- Negative mood states including depression, anxiety and stress (Hopley and Nicki 2010)

Not all of these factors are unique to Internet problem gamblers. Existing literature suggests that problem gambling is more prevalent among younger adults, those
from lower socio-economic groups and people with a family history of problem
gambling (Derevensky and Gupta 2007; Productivity Commission 2010; Reith
2006; Shaffer and Korn 2002; Wardle et al. 2011a). Problem gamblers are also more
likely to gamble on a greater number of gambling activities, have higher gambling
expenditure and longer and more frequent gambling sessions (Productivity
Commission 2010; LaPlante et al. 2009; Wardle et al. 2011a; Welte et al. 2009).
Problem gamblers appear to have a greater number of irrational beliefs, co-morbid
health and psychiatric problems, including addictions and experience dissociation
and negative mood states and be prone to boredom and impulsivity (Gaboury, and
Ladouceur 1989; Petry 2005; Productivity Commission 2010; Wardle et al. 2011a).
However, there does appear to be a discrepancy between Internet problem gamblers
and non-Internet problem gamblers in terms of income and education, which may
be related to the technology required to access Internet gambling.

Characteristics of Self-Excluded Internet Gamblers

Self-exclusion is a process by which individuals enter into an agreement with a
gambling operator that they cannot be allowed to gamble and must be prevented
from making bets. It is typically enacted by individuals in acknowledgment of the
problems that have been caused by their inability to control their gambling resulting
in significant negative consequences.

Analyses of account holders that placed live action bets on a European Internet
gambling site (bwin)found that those who closed their accounts due to gambling-
related problems experienced increasing money loss, increasing stakes per bet, and
increasingly shorter odds bets as the time of account closure approached (Xuan and
Shaffer 2009). This suggests that when self-identified problem gamblers incur
increasing losses they adopt a more risk-aversive, conservative pattern of behaviour
and place higher amounts on bets with lower odds or better chances of winning.

Analysis of this cohort of online sports bettors concentrated on those that had
participated in live action sports betting and closed their account (n=530)
(Braverman and Shaffer 2010). Of these, the majority (92%) were male and the
mean age at time of registration was 28.4. Four clusters of bettors were identified:
(1) gamblers who played frequently and intensively with high variability of wager
size, but increasing value of wagers; (2) gamblers who played very rarely; (3) gamblers who played as frequently as those in (1) and intensively, but bet about the same

amount of money each day that they gambled; and (4) the majority of gamblers who played rarely, not intensively, with low variability in their wager size. The vast majority (73%) of the high activity, high variability cluster reported closing their account due to gambling-related problems, substantially higher rates than for the other clusters, although no demographic details or single variable was associated with closing an account due to gambling problems. Although these results are based on individuals that may not be representative of problem Internet gamblers, they do provide some insight into the behaviour of potentially at-risk gamblers.

Another study surveyed 259 individuals that requested self-exclusion from a European Internet gambling site (Hayer and Meyer 2011). Self-report measures indicated that 68% of respondents had gambling problems. The self-excluders were males, with a mean age of 36.2 years and indicated that Internet casino games were the most problematic, followed by skill games. For 60% of the self-excluders, gambling sessions lasted on average at least 1 h, and 22% reported typically having gambled more than €500 a week on the particular site alone. However, these results must be considered with caution given that only 3% of self-excluders agreed to be included in the study, indicating that the sample may not be representative of problem gamblers.

Furthermore, for both studies participants had self-disclosed gambling problems and requested self-exclusion, an action that is taken by a minority of problem gamblers. For example, in a study of PokerRoom.com, only 3–4% of customers used protection measures such as setting maximum bet/loss restrictions and using self-exclusion (Remmers 2006). Therefore, it is difficult to ascertain the behaviour of those individuals with gambling problems who did not close their accounts due to reported gambling problems.

The use of self-exclusion as a means of limiting gambling-related harms is discussed in further detail in the following chapter. Although evidence is mixed on the extent to which Internet gambling causes problems, it certainly may contribute to and exacerbate problems for vulnerable individuals. Ongoing efforts should focus on ways in which vulnerable populations can be protected and Internet gambling-related harms can be minimised.

Chapter 7
Responsible Gambling Strategies

Abstract Internet gambling poses new challenges to regulators and industry operators in terms of player protection. However, it also offers opportunities through the use of technologically-sophisticated responsible gambling strategies. Internet gambling players can be tracked over time and procedures may be developed that identify potentially risky patterns of play and prompt customers to play within their limits. Online gambling sites may also provide effective time and money limit setting, targeted messaging and education and self-testing options. There is some evidence to indicate that such online tools would be effective at preventing problem gambling and reduce risks of harm. Efforts are also required to prevent harm relating to problem gambling at a wider public health level. For example, restrictions on advertising online gambling sites should be considered, particularly those that may influence youth or are from unregulated sites. This chapter outlines the various responsible gambling strategies that have been implemented on gambling sites and evidence to support the effectiveness of these including player messaging, feedback on gambling behavior, time and money limits, and self-exclusion.

Keywords Internet gambling • Online gaming • Responsible gambling • Harm minimization • Messaging • Limits • Feedback • Self-exclusion • Policy • Customer protection

Responsible gambling refers to the concept of consumer protection (harm-minimization) achieved through attempts to restrict a gambler's expenditure of time and money to within affordable limits (Blaszczynski et al. 2005; Breen et al. 2005; Hing 2004). The premise is based on the assumption that community members choose their levels of involvement but governments and gambling operators retain a duty of care or some measure of responsibility in protecting participants from harm (Blaszczynski et al. 2004; Delfabbro 2008). Internet gamblers cannot be presumed to be representative of the broader population of gamblers and, as highlighted above, Internet gambling has unique features that may be related to harmful consequences.

S. Gainsbury, *Internet Gambling: Current Research Findings and Implications*,
SpringerBriefs in Behavioral Medicine 1, DOI 10.1007/978-1-4614-3390-3_7,
© Springer Science+Business Media, LLC 2012

Subsequently, strategies in place for other types of gambling may not be effective in reducing harm related Internet gambling. Furthermore, minimal evidence has been found to support the effectiveness of responsible gambling initiatives currently in place for land-based gambling, which is not entirely surprising given that the majority of these are not based on empirical evidence, but extrapolated from strategies used in other public health domains such as tobacco and alcohol consumption (Monaghan and Blaszczynski 2010a, b). To effectively protect players from harm and comply with the intentions of responsible gambling policies, it is essential that the design of harm-minimization strategies be based upon theoretically sound principles and empirical support (Monaghan 2009b).

There is some evidence to support consumer demand for effective responsible gambling tools and options. A survey of 10,865 Internet gamblers from 96 countries found that 63% of respondents reported there is 'some' or 'a lot of' need for improvements to responsible gambling features on Internet gambling sites (Gainsbury et al. unpublished manuscript). This is consistent with other sources indicating that the introduction of responsible gambling measures increases favourable attitudes and levels of trust towards gaming operators amongst Internet and non-Internet gamblers (Nisbet 2005; Parke et al. 2008; Schellinck and Schrans 2007; Wood and Griffiths 2008). For example, reports from a self-selected sample of Swedish online poker players indicate that the existence of responsible gambling measures increases levels of trust towards gambling sites by demonstrating corporate integrity and reducing player's anxiety about winning from other players (Wood and Griffiths 2008).

However, despite demand from regulators and customers for effective responsible gambling options, relatively little research has been conducted to guide the implementation of such tools. Furthermore, responsible gambling strategies appear to be of minimal importance to many online gambling operators. In 2004, a study of 30 UK online gambling sites found that 97% did not offer self-exclusion, 77% had no reference to controlled gambling, and 37% had no age verification registration (Smeaton and Griffiths 2004). In a follow-up study of the 20 most popular online gambling sites accessed in Britain, 60% of the websites provided problem gambling information and/or a link to help services websites (Jawad and Griffiths 2008). Only four sites (20%) were given a 'high' rating for the effectiveness of their responsible gambling measures and included measures such as self-assessment tests, daily/weekly deposit limits, options for self-exclusion, and filtering programs. It was noted that most of these options were not located on the sites' home page, but that customers were required to scroll through several pages to find the relevant information (Jawad and Griffiths 2008).

The industry has progressed significantly in recent years, partly due to the increased regulatory requirements and self-imposed operator codes of responsibility, including criteria for third-party endorsements. A study completed by eCOGRA found that the responsible gambling standards of various private gambling operators in Europe were at least as good as, if not better, than some of Europe's leading gambling monopolies (Monaghan 2008). The study revealed that 67% of the consumer-facing standards implemented by members of the EGBA match, or exceed those applied by ten of Europe's largest gambling monopolies. Only 4% of the standards applied by private operators were deemed to be less than those of the monopolies, while 24% exceeded them. These results suggest that private online gambling operators have the capacity to self-regulate their sites and provide suitable player protection and responsible gambling practices. In some cases, the private sector appears to be leading the field in this important area.

Potential Internet-Based Responsible Gambling Measures

By regulating online gambling sites, governments would be able to offer a safer Internet gambling environment (Gainsbury 2010). Early intervention measures may successfully prevent or at least reduce the likelihood of individuals develop gambling-related problems (Tolchard et al. 2006; Petry 2005). Regulations should mandate strict standards for probity and harm-minimization and measures should be tested in advance of and following implementation (Productivity Commission 2010). Currently a variety of responsible gambling measures are being used by online gambling operators and mandated by various jurisdictions. The European Committee for Standardization (2011) agreement contains a whole chapter dedicated to problem gambling prevention measures. Potential measures to protect customers and reduce the harms associated with online gambling include:

- Player identification with multiple forms of identification required to verify identify and address to prevent underage play, duplicate accounts and betting by individuals involved in an event;
- Clear communication of account activity, including losses, in an easily comprehendible and meaningful format;
- Pre-commitment strategies for time and money and automatic bet and deposit limits (per day and month) with an appropriate maximum level and prompts to set lower personal limits;
- Time delays for any increase to time and money limits to reduce chasing of losses and impulsive decisions;
- Periodic reminders and updates of amount lost and time spent playing for individual sessions and longer periods (e.g., weekly) as appropriate;
- Built in pauses and brief breaks in play to prevent dissociation and allow rational decision making;
- Education about games, statistical probabilities of winning and responsible gambling including practical strategies for responsible gambling;
- Feedback on player behaviour including self-tests and alert systems which identify potentially problematic play;
- Self-exclusion options (minimum of 6 months) should be easy to enact. Players should not be contacted during the period or at the end of their self-exclusion;

- Briefer temporary breaks in play should be possible for shorter periods (e.g., 24 h, 7 days) or for certain days (e.g. following receipt of payment/welfare cheques and major sporting events);
- Customer support including referrals to appropriate self-exclusion tools and treatment services;
- Employee training about possible problem gambling and how to identify it;
- Verification that payment methods used belong to account holder;
- A ban on credit betting;
- A limit on the number of credit cards and bank accounts that can be linked to any single account and consistency between where deposits are received from and withdrawals paid to;
- Delays on winnings being paid or re-gambled;
- Links to problem gambling information, support and counselling options.

An example of a responsible approach to online gambling can be seen with Svenska Spel's state owned Internet gambling site in Sweden. This site has many responsible gambling tools to assist players to gamble in a controlled manner. In line with this approach, there are no freerolls, no bonuses and reportedly lower player returns as compared to offshore sites. Before it was launched concerns were expressed that even a highly regulated site could increase gambling problems, that there are few empirical evaluations of the responsible gambling measures, gamblers could still access offshore sites (Stymne 2008). Only moderate advertising is allowed for the site, with no direct links. Other responsible gambling measures include:

- Mandatory limits for the amount of money lost and time played
- Self-exclusion for both short and longer periods
- A self-test for gambling problems that is easily available
- Information on time and money spent that is easily available
- Information about the national help-line and counselling on problem gambling

An evaluation of the site suggests that most gamblers are positive towards the responsible gambling features; however, those playing only at Svenska Spel are more positive than those who also play on other sites and are also have fewer gambling problems (Wood and Griffiths 2008). Svenska Spel may be attracting individuals who want a safe site, although the majority of Swedish players appear to be using offshore online gambling. Of players that reached their pre-set limits, 30% proceeded to gamble on other sites, although this was more likely for at-risk players (Stymne 2008). Similarly, the self-test was used by 16% of all players, but among 24% of at-risk players, indicating some success in encouraging at-risk players to use the responsible gambling tools. The launch of Svenska Spel's poker site corresponded with an increase in the number of Internet poker players; out of 200,000 poker players estimated to exist in 2008, 30,000 started play at Svenska Spel and now play on other sites (Stymne 2008). It is difficult to estimate the success of the responsible gambling tools provided, although at least these are now an option for those that want to use them.

Use of Account Information for Player Interventions and Feedback

The information collected by Internet gambling sites in relation to unique customer accounts provides valuable opportunities to interact with players at a personal level to encourage responsible gambling (Gainsbury 2011). The ability to monitor play and interact and communication with identified players is a key advantage that should be maximised to enable responsible play. For example, information on wins and losses can be clearly and easily displayed for players so they can view their expenditure history. Links can also be provided to help-seeking and information services, including online treatment options, self-help, peer-based discussion forums, and emergency support (Gainsbury and Blaszczynski 2011a). Information from individual accounts, included specific gambling behaviours, can be used to identify potentially risky play, enabling operators to intervene with players as appropriate to minimise risk of harm (Gainsbury 2011). One study of player account behaviour from online gambling operators identified potential behavioural markets of problem gambling that were used to predict future self-exclusion with an accuracy rate of 77% (Haefeli et al. 2011). The markers identified as important factors included a greater frequency of customer services contacts and the tonality (threatening) and subjects (payments, financial transactions, and doubts about the results of games) of the interactions. This one study is an example of the type of research that can be conducted to assist online gambling operators to identify customers that are at risk of harms and may require some sort of intervention to assist them to retain control of their gambling.

Dragicevic et al. (2011) used player account data to analyse online gambling behaviour in attempt to identify risk factors for problem gambling also proposed a conceptual model of how player feedback mechanisms could work. According to this model, player account data should be made available for behaviour analysis, which is undertaken in the context of problem gambling risk factors. The resulting feedback should then be communicated to players, and where appropriate, various responsible gambling tools and features should be made available to players that will assist players in regulating their play. More work is needed to identify behavioural risk factors for online problem gambling, however, collaboration between industry and researchers may make a significant contribution to the field by creating a system that detects risky players enabling early intervention and prevention of gambling problems.

Internet gambling sites should provide gamblers with prominent and easy access to some types of feedback about their problem gambling status (Gainsbury and Blaszczynski 2011b). Online gambling sites should also facilitate self-tests of gambling-related problems that can be easily completed by players and provide automatic normative feedback comparing the individuals' responses to their peers matched by age, gender and culture (Monaghan and Wood 2010). This feedback may make online gambling customers more cognisant of the nature of their gambling behaviours and repeatedly conveyed to individual players so that they can monitor their gambling behaviour over time. Research trials have shown support for the provision of normative feedback to gamblers as a tool to increase awareness of behaviour and increase responsible play, particularly for problem gamblers (Cunningham et al. 2001, 2009; Wood and Williams 2010).

Research indicates that the majority of gamblers would like the option receive feedback on their transactions, such as how much they spend on a given day or month (McDonnell-Phillips 2005). Player feedback indicates that receiving regular financial statements is one of the most popular options for responsible gambling tools, endorsed by 75% of 10,000 respondents in a survey of online gamblers by eCOGRA (2007). In a survey of Swedish online gamblers, 36% of 2,348 participants reported that receiving feedback on their gambling profile in the context of gambling problems was useful (Griffiths et al. 2009b). These results indicate that providing player feedback on their account information in an easy to comprehend and accessible format would be a useful responsible gambling strategy to assist players to gamble within affordable means. However, more research is needed to investigate the impact of this strategy on reducing and preventing problem gambling and also strategies to encourage greater use of such tools by online gamblers.

Pop-Up Messages

The Internet may enable greater communication directly with individual players using measures such as pop-up messages to capture attention and deliver meaningful, tailored messages (Monaghan 2009b; Monaghan and Blaszczynski 2010a). It has been proposed that pop-up messages may effectively increase responsible gambling and reduce the incidence of problem gambling on Internet gambling sites (Monaghan 2009b). This is based on findings that pop-up messages appearing on EGM screens during a short break in play were associated with more breaks in play, shorter sessions, and an increased reported impact on thoughts and behaviours than standard static messages (Monaghan and Blaszczynski 2010a). Pop-up messages have also been successfully demonstrated to increase adherence to time and money limits amongst gamblers as they broke dissociation and enabled players to focus on their gambling (Wohl and Pellizzari 2011). Pop-up messages that appear on player's screens at regular intervals may be useful in disrupting playing and any potential dissociation, thereby helping players become more aware of their behaviour (including time and money spent gambling). This should enable players to make more informed decisions and to gamble in a more responsible manner. Studies of Internet pop-ups advertisements show that when pop-ups are displayed when the user's cognitive effort is low and are perceived as relevant, valuable and contain useful information, they elicit less irritation and avoidance (Edwards et al. 2002; Pasadeos 1990). These results are confirmed by in-venue studies which report that pop-up messages and short breaks in play do not overly disturb gamblers and are viewed favourably as a responsible gambling strategy by a substantial proportion of gamblers (Monaghan and Blaszczynski 2010a; Rodda and Cowie 2005). Therefore, pop-up messages causing a short break in play that contain useful and relevant information, such as updates on time and money spent, should not disturb recreational Internet gamblers and may be an effective responsible gambling strategy (Monaghan 2009b).

Time and Money Limits

Given that time and money spent gambling and the number of gambling sessions are predictive of an Internet gambler experiencing gambling problems, online gambling sites should introduce limits that assist players to control their gambling to reasonable and affordable levels. Research suggests that the majority of gamblers, including problem gamblers, have tried to self-regulate by having some kind of spending limit in mind (McDonnell-Phillips 2005). Players are also generally in favour of having option to set their own limits when gambling. In an empirical study, young adult recreational gamblers were shown an animation about how outcomes are determined that attempted to reduce irrational beliefs. Of those that saw the animation, 94% of participants stayed within their set time limit, compared to only 67% of those that did not see the animation. Pop-up messages reminding players to set a time limit achieved the same adherence, within even less disruption to play (Wohl and Pellizzari 2011), indicating that a simple strategy of asking players to set a limit can be highly useful. The addition of a pop-up message reminding players when they have reached their limit further reduces gambling play and expenditure and increases the proportion of participants that gamble within their affordable limits. However, as these studies were conducted with university students provided with credit to gamble, the results require further testing in actual online gambling sites and with players who are at greater risk of harm. When gamblers were asked whether they thought that tools to set time and monetary limits would be useful, these were highly endorsed by players as options that should be provided by online operators (Wohl and Pellizzari 2011).

Many online gambling sites currently offer players the opportunity to set limits on their gambling behaviour. For example, Sportsbet.com, one of Australia's leading online betting sites (owned by Paddy Power with over 750,000 registered and 200,000 active customers), allows customers to voluntarily place deposits limits on how much they are willing to spend on a daily, weekly or monthly basis, which cannot be changed for 60 days. In a statement to the Australian Senate Gambling Reform Committee, Mr. Cormac Benedict, Sportsbet CEO stated that 1,600 customers had set deposit limits. This indicates that voluntary tools may only be used by a minority of customers. Higher usage was reported in relation to Betfair Australia, who reported that approximately 12,000 customers (out of 100,000 active customers) had utilised loss limits, although changes could be made after 7 days to relax previously set limits. This indicates that there is some demand amongst online gamblers for limit setting tools.

Broda and colleagues (2008) conducted a study of gambling behaviour of 47,000 members of an Internet sports betting service provider, bwin, which imposes limits on the amount of money users can deposit into their online gambling accounts. Analysis of the data revealed that a very small proportion of players (0.3%) exceeded the deposit limits at least once. However, pre-set deposit limits are very high and only prevent users from depositing more than €1,000 per 24 h, or €5,000 per 30 days. The vast majority of users (99.7%) in Broda et al. (2008) study never deposited more than €500 per 24 h and never deposited more than €1,050 per 30 days, indicating that deposit limits could be substantially lowered without impacting the majority of customers. Individuals who exceeded deposit limits had a greater betting frequency and higher average bet size than gamblers not exceeding deposit limits. Those who exceeded limits received an average of 14 messages (SD = 29, Median = 6) and continued to wager in a manner suggesting that the feedback about a violation of policy failed to have the intended harm-minimization impact.

In an examination of the same sample of bwin users, 1.2% of individuals chose to impose self-limits, which ranged from €9-€4,177. Although the majority of these users made only the initial change, 12.2% made multiple changes (Nelson et al. 2008). Only 7.1% of individuals initially placed self-limits and the average duration from the first bet to self-imposition of limits was 213 days, suggesting this may be a strategy used to limit play due to the experience of negative consequences related to excessive online play. Following self-imposition of limits, individuals generally decreased their bet size and frequency, although total amount wagered did not change significantly. Over 10% of these users ceased all betting on bwin after imposing self-limits, suggesting this feature may have assisted them to reconsider their gambling behaviour or switch to an alternate site.

In a study that included player behaviour over several sites, but was limited to a sample recruited from Sweden, it was found that when the set limit was reached on Svenska Spel's online poker site, 30% of all players gambled on alternate sites, with 50% of risk-players continuing to gamble on other sites (Stymne 2008). This highlights the difficulties of enforcing limits in an attempt to encourage responsible gambling as players can easily switch to other sites. However, it also demonstrates that the majority of players who reached limits did cease to gamble, suggesting that these measures may be effective in facilitating responsible play for certain individuals. At the very least it provides a cool-down period for the gambler although it may not be economically profitable for the gambling site.

If limits are to be used as a responsible gambling feature by online gambling sites, they should be sufficiently low as to avert potential problems that seem to arise from excessive gambling. For example, the pre-set limits on bwin (reported above) and similarly the CAD$9,999 weekly limit on British Columbia's *Play Now* are artificially high and unlikely to prevent any problems. Analysis of player behaviour will enable operators to estimate typical gambling expenditure in terms of time and money and provide various levels of prompts for appropriate limits to encourage responsible levels of play.

Self-Exclusion

One of the many available measures used to minimise gambling-related harms is the option of self-exclusion. Formal exclusion programs are also used in land-based venues and are designed to prevent individuals from accessing gambling facilities. These programs are typically used by individuals who have difficulty controlling their gambling and are experiencing problems and use self-exclusion as an external support in their efforts to abstain from gambling (Hayer and Meyer 2011). A study of 259 individuals that requested self-exclusion from a European Internet gambling site found that 27% of the participants had use online self-exclusion options previously (Hayer and Meyer 2011). Follow-up surveys with 20 respondents suggest that the temporary restriction of access to one single online gambling site had favourable psycho-social effects, including a reduction in problem gambling. It should also be noted that problem gambling is not the only reason that players choose to self-exclude from gambling sites; prevention and annoyance with the site were also motivators for self-exclusion.

Swedish state operator Svenska Spel has implemented many optional measures designed to promote responsible gambling such as self-tests, self-set limits for time and money, and self-exclusion (Jonsson 2008). This site offers a voluntary player tracking system known as 'PlayScan' that is designed to inform players when their gambling behaviour changes in such a way that might suggest it is becoming problematic. In an online survey of 1,031 randomly selected Svenska Spel poker players, only 5.4% of respondents confirmed having used the self-exclusion option at least once, which represents 11% of at-risk players (Jonsson 2008). During the exclusion period, 30% of this group played on other poker sites and continued to gamble there. A survey of 2,348 Svenska Spel customers, reported that 26% of respondents had used the responsible gambling tools, and 52% of these participants stated that they found it useful, compared to 19% that reported they did not find it useful (Griffiths et al. 2009b). Participants reported being primarily motivated by a desire to save money and address excessive gambling.

As the respondents for these studies self-selected to participate in the survey, they may not be representative of the wider population of online gamblers. However, evidence from the Australian betting websites indicates that only a minority of customers use self-exclusion options. In a statement to the Senate Gambling Reform Committee interactive gambling inquiry in August 2011, the CEO of Sportsbet, Mr. Barry, stated that out of 750,000 registered and 200,000 active customers, only 900 had self-excluded. In the same inquiry, Mr. Blanksby, Legal Director for Betfair Australia stated that out of the approximate 200,000 Australian customers, around 2,500 had self-excluded.

A significant limitation of this method of harm-minimisation is the lack of collaboration between different online gambling sites and venues, so that excluded individuals may find it easy to gamble at another site or venue. However, the technological capabilities of Internet gambling means that it may be possible for online gambling operators to share data to support more innovative harm-minimisation approaches, such as cross-operator self-exclusion (Dragicevic 2011). For example, it is a UK licensing condition to maintain a register of self-excluders, including appropriate records of identification details and payment cards. Although care must be taken to protect customer identity, data encryption programs can be used to protect sensitive details and it may be possible to encourage operators to share details to enable wider self-exclusion programs. One program, VerPlay.org has been developed by Bet Buddy that allows safe and secure exchange of anonymous operator data that would allow operators to check whether their players are on the central list of self-excluded players (Dragicevic 2011). This collaborative effort would help protect vulnerable gamblers, although regulatory efforts may be required to prompt operators to enact such measures.

Central Agency for Responsible Gambling

As online gamblers may hold multiple accounts with a variety of operators, responsible gambling systems may be made much more efficient if data is shared between operators and regulators. Operators may be concerned that if they take actions to assist customers that may be at risk of having problems, the customer may just move to another site and continue to gamble. A centralised agency may be established at a country, regional or international level that collects data on clients that meet certain parameters, such as extremely frequent betting, high bet sizes, and high losses, to be determined based on empirical research. The centralised agency could assist all gambling operators to take a cohesive approach to minimising gambling-related harms.

A centralised agency would also establish self-exclusion across a range of online gambling sites and operators to provide a more effective self-exclusion program for customers experiencing gambling-related harms. Self-exclusion with individual online operators is obviously limited in that there are numerous alternative options for gamblers. A central agency may ensure that all operators check the identity of customers and exclude those that require assistance in controlling their gambling. Licensing rights within a particular jurisdiction may require gambling operators to implement this cooperative strategy to protect players from harm. Efforts should also be undertaken to create international standards and agreements to avoid players using offshore sites to avoid self-exclusion policies enacted on onshore sites (Productivity Commission 2010). However, it is acknowledged that such cooperation could not be mandatory or complete and problem gamblers are likely to always be able to access some online gambling sites should they choose to do so.

An existing example of a secure service for managing self-exclusion across operators is VeriPlay, powered by Bet Buddy. VeriPlay aims to act as an intermediary to assist online gambling operators to more effectively use their player data to protect vulnerable players. The system will maintain a centralised database of self-excluded players, whose details are safely and securely stored using anonymised player data and encryption algorithms. Operators can add self-excluded players and check whether new or existing players should be excluded. The adoption of such a system by an operator would strengthen their compliance with responsible gambling policies and processes.

Chapter 8
Future Trends

Abstract Internet gambling will continue to evolve in response to consumer demand, market developments, political and regulatory changes and technological advances. Participation and revenue appear to be increasing as more individuals and groups use this mode of gambling. It is likely that more jurisdictions will liberalise Internet gambling in recognition of the difficulties with prohibition, the importance of providing a safe playing environment and economic benefits. Reputation, branding, marketing, security and customer interaction will continue to be vital for online gambling sites to be competitive in addition to novel and exciting product. In particular, social media will play an increasing role in Internet gambling. The relationship with sports and sports betting will continue, and Internet gambling operators will increasingly target a wider range of target audiences. Mobile gambling will increase and play an important role. Regulators will have to pay attention to this form of gambling and implement policies to protect individuals, including responsible gambling and prevention strategies and treatment options. This chapter outlines the future trends predicted for online gambling, including the impacts on related industries including land-based gambling and social media.

Keywords Internet gambling • Online gaming • Mobile gambling • Social media • Trends • Predictions • Market drivers • Developments • Consolidation • Gaming

The global outlook suggest continued growth and player migration to online gambling, with Internet gambling revenue rising at 12.1% compounded annually, compared with 2.6% for land-based gambling (PWC 2010). Land-based gambling is predicted to account for the dominate proportion of the global gambling market for many years to come, although Internet gambling will represent an increasing proportion of the global gambling market. Industry reports predict online wagering to show significant continued growth given the similarities between offline and online products and the increased ease and convenience of online betting (Church-Sanders 2011). Compared with other forms of online gambling, sports and race wagering

S. Gainsbury, *Internet Gambling: Current Research Findings and Implications*, 115
SpringerBriefs in Behavioral Medicine 1, DOI 10.1007/978-1-4614-3390-3_8,
© Springer Science+Business Media, LLC 2012

sites have the most effective way to recruit customers through cross-selling and lower cost per customer acquisition (Church-Sanders 2011). Globally the online casino market is also showing huge potential for growth due to its entertainment factor and is predicted to grow in any markets, particularly where the regulatory position is favourable to games of chance (Church-Sanders 2010). However, potential barriers to future developments include economic downturn, lack of infrastructure, payment crackdowns, restrictive legislation and increased competition from other forms of gambling.

Although the rate of growth in new player sign-ups in any individual jurisdiction may decline over time as the market matures, the impact on overall growth will be mitigated by the opening of new foreign markets through increased penetration of broadband and recognition by governments of the need for a proper regulatory framework for online gambling (Church-Sanders 2010). Changing regulatory policies are also likely to affect online sites, particularly sites that defy policies of prohibition if these are increasingly enforced. Furthermore, if prohibited markets do open, there may be preference for legalised sites, who may also receive advantages in terms of endorsements and advertising rights. The fragmented regulatory landscape and various speeds at which regulation is changing in different jurisdictions makes it difficult to predict the future for Internet gambling, although some trends are apparent.

Consolidation

As has been an apparent trend over the past few years, the total number of online gambling sites will remain relatively stable and the number of new sites will reduce. Existing operators are looking to expand in terms of product offerings and will look to move into new foreign markets. The Internet gambling market is highly competitive and overheads must be very low to allow high player payback and bonuses to remain attractive to new and existing customers (Church-Sanders 2010). Sites that do not have sufficient capital to attract and retain customers will not be able to compete with larger operators and a fewer players reduces liquidity, and makes it even more difficult to run a successful gambling site. Competition is likely to increase the quality of the products offered as well as customer service, marketing and branding in an attempt to acquire and retain customers.

The past few years have seen a period of consolidation in the online gambling industry, which is likely to continue. Mergers and acquisitions have occurred between companies that offer similar and different products as a result of efforts both to expand and eliminate the competition. Consolidation is often responsible for the development of strong brands as merged companies are able to offer existing and new customers an increased choice of products and services and continue working with an expert team on new product developments. Mergers and acquisitions may also be driven by a need to expand and acquire expertise, technology and products not currently offered or under-developed. This type of action has seen online sports books expand into online casinos and casinos offer poker rooms and so forth. For example, in March 2011, PartyGaming and bwin completed a merger. In some cases, larger operators will simply buy smaller sites and operators to reduce competition and increase market share. Successful operators are also using public offerings to acquire capital that may be used to facilitate expansion through acquisitions.

Gaming law expert, I. Nelson Rose (2010) confirms that by purchasing an established brand name site or event, like the World Series of Poker, an operator can acquire substantial marketing power. He highlights the similarity between the current trend in the online gambling field to that which has occurred between land-based operators, resulting in large multinational companies commanding a significant proportion of the casino gambling market. However, unlike land-based casinos, online operations can be transferred and modified much more quickly and easily. Online operators can finalise deals and transfers in less than a year and with much less disruption to operations and customers. Furthermore, less capital may be caught in online gambling sites compared to large commercial properties, meaning that more cash may be available for acquisitions by online operators. As the online gambling industry continues to grow, it is expected that the period of consolidation will continue and large, global brands will begin to dominate certain markets and offer a variety of products to satisfy a range of customers.

Existing Gambling Companies Entering the Online Gambling Market

Existing gambling operators are increasingly recognizing the importance of online gambling as a means to diversify existing product offerings and capture further market share. Online gambling can be offered in addition to existing land-based gambling activities in an attempt to generate substantial revenues that have been realized by existing online gambling operators. Online gambling can also be used to direct customers into land-based venues, for example, by hosting poker tournaments in venues, offering bonuses for online play that can only be redeemed in venues or other marketing promotions (Gros 2011b). Existing player loyalty schemes can also be extended to cover both online and land-based gambling to create a harmonious system. This may be useful in particular for destination casinos to maintain customer engagement in between visits and increase the likelihood of customers returning to venues.

There has been some opposition from existing land-based operators to Internet gambling, partially due to concerns about cannibalization of revenue streams and a lack of fair regulation across the modes. The powerful US lobby group, the AGA, which represents a substantial proportion of the US casino industry opposed liberalization of online gambling for many years (Vardi 2011). However, in March 2010, the AGA board reversed this decision and the group now supports online gambling regulation, starting with online poker, which has had substantial impacts in terms of political movement and lobbying efforts (Vardi 2011). The ability of existing gambling companies to move online in part depends on the regulation in the markets they currently exist in as well as their ability to penetrate foreign markets. Although casino groups are currently limited to lobbying, in Australia, wagering company Tabcorp reported that the Internet accounted for more than 10% of the value of all best wagered in 2009 and online wagering increased 18% in the first half of the financial year of 2009 ('PaddyPower buys into Australia' 2010). Other Australian bookmakers are reporting strong growth online ('PaddyPower buys into Australia' 2010). Caesars Entertainment (formerly Harrah's) has successfully moved into the online market now offering casino, bingo and poker products (Church-Sanders 2010), although only in jurisdictions in which online gambling is permitted, which obviously excludes the US.

Many casino operations already have established brand names/recognition, which may help them quickly become dominant players in the online gambling market. Their reputations may allow for the transference of existing beliefs about a physical entity to a virtual entity (Coltman et al. 2001). Existing gambling operators have substantial databases with contact details for all patrons and can offer a variety of bonuses and rewards for players. For example, when the MGM/Mirage opened an online casino operating from the Isle of Man, 60% of its registration attempts were from customers in the US (Hornbuckle 2003). However, initially acquiring loyal customers and being able to sustain customers while acquiring new consumers is difficult for online gambling operators. This has been seen, for example when 2 years after establishing online gambling portals licensed in the Isle of Man, two strong gambling brands, MGM/Mirage and Sun International, abandoned their online gambling operations, citing high operating costs in the highly regulated environment and the difficulty of competing against relatively unregulated Caribbean-based operations. Similarly, the Australian owners of Crown Casino in Melbourne relinquished its Vanuatu-based online casino operations in 2003 due to a lack of success (Eadington 2004). This highlights the difficulties in operating successful Internet gambling sites as compared to land-based venues, which often have a more captive customer base and less competition.

It is now somewhat difficult for some land-based brands to enter the market and compete with established Internet gambling companies which, through heavy advertising and publicity, have already achieved brand recognition. Jurisdictions that offer a closed market or monopoly may have more success due to the reduced legal competition from other operators. It is difficult for land-based operators to watch offshore sites directly target customers when they are legally not allowed to offer online gambling themselves; however, caution is needed in forming partnerships or purchasing offshore operators, which may reduce their ability to offer online gambling products if regulation changes.

Several slot machine manufactures, including International Game Technology (IGT), Bally, and WMS have entered the online sector and transformed successful land-based products into online games. IGT purchased Entraction Holding AB from Sweden, which has one of the world's largest online poker networks and is one of the leading suppliers to the industry (Rose 2011). This was a clear use of mergers and acquisitions to gain instant expertise, while retaining credibility as the company had never taken bets from the US that may cause future difficulties with regulators. Australian-based Aristocrat Leisure has signed a contract with Maryland Live! Casino, a new gaming and entertainment destination, to launch a play-for-fun online casino ('Aristocrat secures first online deal' 2011). This will be the first property to integrate Aristocrat's online system, nLive, and the online free-play casino will launch in March 2012 ahead of the land-based casino's grant opening. The online casino site will include poker, slots and skill-based games and allow Maryland Live! to log-on line and earn reward points in the online casino to build the land-based casino's brand, market to new and existing customers, establish customer relations and encourage players back to the land-based casino. Aristocrat has made a similar arrangement with Michigan-based Island Resort & Casino ('Second U.S casino to go online' 2011). By launching a free-play online casino a land-based venue may be well-placed to offer online gambling should regulations be changed in the US.

Other land-based casinos have also taken steps to be involved in the online gambling market internationally and in the US should regulation be changed. Caesar's Interactive Entertainment, a subsidiary of Caesars Entertainment has a partnership with 888 Holdings and is reportedly considered a strategic partnership to operate online poker once the it is legalized (Rose 2011). Wynn Resorts entered into an alliance with PokerStars, in March 2011, in a strategic relationship to work towards legalization and regulation of poker in the US and position Wynn as a leading online poker operator in the event of legalisation. However, this partnership was swiftly ended following the prosecutorial actions from the US in April, 2011. Nonetheless, it is expected that existing land-based gambling operators will continue to consider the online gambling market as an important area for future investment.

Existing Non-Gambling Companies Entering the Market

Large, non-gambling companies are recognizing the potential revenues associated with Internet gambling and the need to diversify their own product offerings. Companies that are well placed to move into the online gambling field are those with an existing customer base and online presence, such as media owners and online game operators. Operators that have existing expertise in customer management, including analyzing customer behavior and providing individualized feedback, as well as those with existing marketing and technology are more likely to be successful (Church-Sanders 2010).

Online gaming companies are entering the online gambling market. Virgin Gaming has signed a deal with Electronic Arts to support many of its popular sports video games, using its online wagering system (Pilieci 2011). This will allow video gamers to wager on the outcomes of their own video game challenges and in gaming tournaments. Similarly, online gaming and entertainment company 2UP Gaming has entered into an agreement to purchase an online casino affiliate business that provides links to Internet gambling services ('Online gaming and entertainment' 2011).

2UP managing director stated that the purchase was a strategic move to provide immediate cash flow to the company and eventually move to becoming a major international online gambling company.

There are many similarities between online gaming and gambling, although companies offering games will be challenged to modify existing products to create new revenue, in particular where they are locked to a particular platform. For example, Zynga, which operates the highly popular and profitable FarmVille and Zynga Poker amongst other games, is locked in a deal with Facebook in which it must use Facebook credits as currency. This can be considered a form of social gaming, which is likely to provide a platform to open gaming to a wider audience of players that would not typically consider themselves as gamblers, but may cross-over into an online gambling site.

Media companies are already starting to offer online games to customers in an effort to gather micropayments as an ongoing source of revenue. For example, Australian online readers of the Daily Telegraph will be charged around AUD$1.50 to play trivia games against other players for prize money ('News Ltd' 2009). Moves have already been made to offer online betting products to media readers; In August 2011, Soccer Millionaire, the UK and Alderney licensed online games developer, signed an online gaming supply deal with the UK's Daily Telegraph newspaper ('The Daily Telegraph' 2011). The agreement will see Soccer Millionaire continue to provide pool betting products and skill games to the UK newspaper's Fantasy Football offering in addition to providing online casino games to The Daily Telegraph for the first time.

As with the discussion of mergers and acquisitions above, entry into the online gambling market is not easy and competition between sites is very strong. In some cases, non-gambling companies may look to the Internet gambling industry for revenue through the provision of non-gambling services. For example, in 2009, Australia Post entered into an agreement with leading Australian betting provider, Tabcorp, in which customers could access over-the-counter services at Australia Post outlets. Although they will not directly facilitate betting services, Australia Post can conduct identity verification procedures, accept new account applications and facilitate deposits, withdrawals and balance information. Such options may be more appealing for businesses located in jurisdictions where regulatory direction and policies limit the extent to which non-gambling brands can actively pursue this market. Given the continued growth expected for online gambling, it is expected that interest in entering this market will continue from outside the industry.

Targeting New Markets

As the online gambling market matures, existing and new operators must target new markets by moving into foreign jurisdictions and capturing non-traditional gamblers. Acquisition of customers in foreign jurisdictions is partially dependent on broadband and mobile penetration and regulatory policies. Previous sections of this book have discussed new and emerging markets internationally in terms of regulatory change and potential for revenue. Opening of new foreign markets will have considerable impacts on the industry, although regulatory changes are somewhat unpredictable in the online gambling field. Asia and India have a growing middle class with more wealth in general and strong Internet and particularly mobile connections. A study published by the Media Entertainment Consulting Network identified the new market in India and Asia as the fastest growing area for online wagering products ('India and Asia new ground for online casino operators' 2011). Subsequently, these markets have attracted attention from international operators.

In some foreign jurisdictions, partnership with local companies is often desirable, both to meet regulatory requirements in some cases and to provide local and culturally-relevant knowledge to ensure relevant products are offered and cultural factors are addressed. Game preferences and platforms for use differ between cultures and jurisdictions. Furthermore, to successfully market products in multiple cultures requires subtle changes. Companies must be able to identify all the nuances that make the different markets unique and reflect these in their sites, from the advertising they are able to employ to the location and that nationality of their sales and customer service support team (Doyle 2008). For example, although the US and UK share a similar language, there are cultural differences which necessitate being addressed (most notably in the area of the types of sporting events). Given that most online gaming companies target wide range of markets it follows they would have employees from a wide range of nationalities (Doyle 2008).

The increasing variety in terms of player demographics has been discussed. The online gambling market increasingly includes women, younger and older customers and players looking for novel forms of entertainment from a safe, secure and trustworthy operator. A workshop held by the European Commission (2011b) concluded that new markets of Internet gamblers are developing in Europe and existing ones are expanding, including young people, women and ethnic minorities. A longitudinal study conducted in Sweden compared Internet gamblers that first played online in 2009 to those who gambled online in previous years (Svensson and Romild 2011). Results found that recent adopters were more likely to be young (less than 40), with low levels of education, and that the gap between men and women in terms of the proportion of online gamblers had decreased over time. In particular, women in relationships with children were more likely than other groups of women to start gambling online and single men with children were also more likely to start online gambling. This suggests that housebound women, and potentially men, may start gambling online due to the availability of this form of gambling. New Internet gamblers appeared to have a history of gambling on land-based forms, including poker, casino gambling, sports betting and lottery, suggesting that gamblers migrated to online play, rather than taking up gambling for the first time.

Online gambling operators may experiment with marketing strategies and use a combination of approaches to recruit players from more traditional markets, such as sports fans and young men, but also create advertisements, marketing strategies and products that appeal to other demographics. Marketing indicatives are increasingly using a combination of traditional deposit, referral and reactivation bonuses as well as non-gaming incentives such as tickets to major events, promotional items and credits for non-gaming activities or prizes. These efforts are generally an attempt to convert non-Internet gamblers into customers and may encourage existing customers to refer their friends and family to sites. Products that appeal to niche demographics and interest are relatively easy to generate online through repackaging of existing games. For example, following the recent popularity of vampire-themed movies and television shows, online slots with vampire-themes and graphics have become available for players. It is difficult to predict the future markets for online gambling, but as the mode continues to increase in popularity it is expected that the customer base will continue to diversify which may challenge operators to widen their offerings, and provide opportunities for smaller operators to find niches.

New Products and Games

Internet gambling sites are increasingly offering a variety of games and products in addition to traditional core products. Offering a greater number of products aims to increase the likelihood of players remaining on a single site, rather than playing on a competitor's site, and therefore spending more time and money and interacting with a single operator longer (Church-Sanders 2010). According to iGaming Business, a typical online gambling operator with a full portfolio of gambling products will obtain around 30% of its revenue from casino games, 40% from betting, 20% from poker, 8% from bingo and 2% from skill games (Church-Sanders 2011). Online operators are challenged to achieve a balance between their core product and side games to avoid cannibalizing their own customer base (Church-Sanders 2011), through customers spending more than they can afford and leaving the site. Online gambling operators must decide whether they will diversify their own expertise to offer additional products, or use another provider for these products. It is important for operators to ensure that all products offered are of a high quality to avoid players being frustrated and leaving a site entirely. As mentioned above, mergers and acquisitions are a common way for an online gambling operator to acquire the necessary experience and platforms to expand their gambling products. Products that are cross-sold to encourage participation in various games may increase profits. For example, sports betting customers may receive bonus credits that must be spend on casino games in an effort to encourage customers to try a variety of games and increase site engagement.

Online gambling options may also become more interactive and have increased entertainment value. For example, online betting sites are increasingly integrating videos into sites to fill the gap between events and also to allow players to watch past performances before making bets. These features are also available via mobile and wireless platforms (e.g., tablets) and digital televisions. In a recent example, the sportsman media group has acquired the live streaming rights to the Australian Open following a 2-year deal with Tennis Australia ('Sportsman addes Australian Open' 2011). This will enable sportsman to add this event to its portfolio of live streaming sports available to its online betting platforms in an effort to enrich live betting for its clients, which include bet365, Betfair, bwin, Interwetten, Bet-at-home, Betclic, Expekt, and Unibet. Gambling operators that provide customers with information to assist them to place bets may be more appealing to novice bettors as well as skilled customers that wish to make informed bets. Increased interaction with customers is also likely to enhance the player's experience on the site, which may increase customer loyalty. A variety of levels of social interaction and features are also being provided to cater to various player demands and receive feedback from players that can drive further relevant developments.

Similarly to online betting, casino games and slots may become more interactive using video clips, social interaction features and characteristics similar to online games. Cross-branding with popular movies and television shows may attract new customers and increase the entertainment value of these sites. Graphics are becoming more sophisticated and players can customize their persona or avatar for a more personalized experience. Betting products are also becoming more varied to include those that can be used for a short time period, or engage a user for extended periods of time, such as tournaments.

Social Networks and Games

The ever increasing popularity and global use of social media and social gaming, and revenue associated with these platforms, suggests that online gambling providers may increasingly look to social media for player attainment and interaction. There are two main categories of social media; social networks, such as Facebook and Twitter that provide a forum for social interaction, content sharing and discussions, and social games, which allow players to interact with one another, see how their friends are doing, and success is typically facilitated by peer-to-peer engagement and competition. Facebook is the most popular social media platform, with over 10% market penetration globally, nearly 50% in North America, 36% in Australia, 26% in Europe, and 21% in Latin America (Miniwatts Marketing Group 2011b). Globally, total active usage of all social networking sites has risen dramatically in all age segments; among those aged 16–24, penetration levels of social networking sites grew 26% from July 2009 to June 3 2011, 46% among those aged 25–34, 35% among those aged 35–44, and 52% among those age 45–54 ('Microblogging' 2011). These figures clearly demonstrate the relevance of social networking to online gambling operators, given the extent of the population that engages with these platforms. There is also evidence of positive engagement with businesses, a deviation from the original purpose of connecting purely socially, as joining a branded group (i.e., 'liking' a Facebook business page), was one of the fastest growing activities on Facebook between July 2009 and June 2011, increasing by 6%.

Both social media platforms typically use virtual currency. For example, Facebook credits are used on social networks and in games on this platform.

Although in theory virtual credits not equivalent to real currencies, black markets have emerged and these are traded for real money. Players can earn, buy, trade and win credits to progress in games. Social games are similar to online gambling in some ways, however, they typically do not monetize in the same way. Social games are often free to play, however they generate revenue through micro-transactions for the sale of virtual goods, and in some cases pay-to-play or subscription-based content for all of some features. In some social games, Zynga's Poker being an obvious example, players can wager virtual currency in gambling-type games, although the credits are not paid out as winnings and anything given to players cannot have monetary value, making these games exempt from gambling regulations.

There are currently a vast variety of free-play gambling opportunities on social networking platforms. An analysis conducted in 2010 found that Facebook had 23 gambling, 338 poker, 16 sports betting, 116 casino and 81 slot apps (Korn et al. 2010). In addition, there were over 2,500 gambling poker, casino, slot and sports betting pages, groups, applications and events providing indirect gambling opportunities, including links to external sites. Gambling operators are increasingly using social media to advertise and recruit players as part of their marketing strategy (Church-Sanders 2011). They are also launching social games to build communities and interact with customers and potential customers, including those in jurisdictions in which they may not be able to operate money games. For example, MGM Resorts International are expected to announce a new social media game, similar to Zynga's FarmVille, in which players pretend to be casino moguls (Berzon 2011).

Free play games with virtual currency allow players to try new games and are already offered by many online gambling operators. Some operators may provide player rewards such as prizes for free play games based on accumulated points. For example, ESPN's "Streak for Cash" sports prediction game offers a monthly grand prize of $50,000, and reportedly has over three million players per day, generating millions for the company (Taylor 2010). Social gaming customers are a suitable market for online gambling operators given the apparent cross-over between the markets; reports indicate that 40% of social game customers have a college degree or higher education attainment, 25% are in a professional or managerial role at work and 55% have a household income of US$50,000 or more (Taylor 2010). Recent moves from Betfair, Caesars Entertainment and PokerStars to invest in social media platforms and companies suggest that social gaming and social networks will play an important role in online gambling in the future.

What remains to be seen is whether social games will be used by online gambling companies for marketing and player engagement or become revenue raisers in their own right. Although some cross-over may occur as players are converted from playing free social games to betting, however, this may not be the ultimate aim and only benefit of such games for operators. Social games can be standalone revenue streams and form part of a larger brand. Users can be encouraged to interact with each other, and the operator, contributing to player understanding and engagement. Most social games rely on traditional advertising models, although other revenue-raising strategies are in place. These include encouraging social gamers to purchase virtual goods to enhance their gaming experience and implementing in-game advertising and sponsorship (Taylor 2010). However, significant revenues linked directly to social gaming have yet to be seen on a grand scale (Bennett 2011c).

The notable exception to this is Zynga, which is valued at US$15 billion to US$20 billion (Wingfield et al. 2011). As of July 2011, Zynga's games on Facebook have over 232 million monthly active users, are some of the most widely used game applications on Facebook and one game, CityVille, has over 14 million daily users ('Form S-1' 2011; Glasser 2011). Texas HoldEm is one of Zynga's oldest and more popular games and has generated significant revenue. It still has 6.95 million daily active users and 36.9 million monthly active users (Eldon 2011), clearly demonstrating the popularity of this type of social game. In a recent UK court case, a hacker was found guilty and faced a substantial prison sentence after stealing Zynga poker chips (Charif 2011). The hacker sold the virtual chips for approximately £50,000 and Zynga valued these chips at $12 million, suggesting that the virtual currency does have real monetary value, and are worthy of protection.

Creating a popular social game is a difficult task, but gambling operators can easily create a social media presence through a Facebook page and Twitter account to interact with new and existing customers. Social networks allow players to reach content easily making gambling operators potentially more accessible to potential customers who do not have to download any software or visit an external site. Ideally social network pages should link customers to gambling sites and loyalty programs, allow customers to interact with the operator to provide feedback and seek responses, and enable players to interact with each other (Flood 2011). Social media engagement should not be thought of as a single marketing campaign, but part of larger customer engagement and should be run by a qualified individual to ensure that it is updated regularly. Cultivation and growth of followers on any social media platform requires a "community manager" to encourage people to join continually, engage participants in a dialogue, and to retain members (Flood 2011). The use of social network by businesses should increase brand awareness, drive new users to the target site, create an engagement loop and access to an open communication channel.

Recent changes to Facebook's advertising policies now allow online gambling operators to advertise directly to users, provided that they are approved and target users over the legal age of 18 within countries where gambling is permitted (Constine 2011). However, gambling advertisements can only be purchased through a direct sales partnership, which requires a minimum monthly spend of US$30,000, and may not be purchased through the self-serve ads tool, indicating that some level of scrutiny may still apply. Nonetheless, whereas operators were previously unable to run promotional ads deemed to encourage gambling, this approach appears to have been significantly softened. Previously, promotions offering free credits or bets, such as "get a $20 free bet" would have to read "get a $20 free bet when you bet $80". Gambling operators were also unable to direct users to online gambling sites, had a limit of four posts a week and content was restricted, deterring the use of Facebook as a marketing channel. Operators can now post content without limits on the frequency of subject opening Facebook as a much more viable means of marketing and communicating with customers and potential customers. The shift in Facebook's advertising policy means that traffic can now be directed from Facebook to a gambling site, making the popular social networking site extremely valuable (Donoghue and Healy 2011). Research indicates that driving traffic to a Facebook brand page is cheaper than driving traffic to an external website, suggesting that this marketing route will be significantly cheaper and potentially more effective given the huge proportion of the population that already use Facebook.

There are a variety of social media platforms beyond Facebook:

- LinkedIn is a social networking site with over 100 million users for the online business community that combines business networking, communication between organizations and companies, and online job hunting. It is based on the premise of shared connections between colleagues and networking groups to communicate information and updates. Online gambling advertising is not directly allowed, although there are several groups specifically catering to the online gambling industry.
- Twitter has over 400 million users and is heavily used for global communication. Users make short posts to their followers making it ideal for brief information sharing and updates.
- Qzone has over 480 million users and is China's biggest social networking site. Gambling advertising is not allowed, although given the potential for China to be a significant market for online gambling in the future, it is potentially important for operators.
- Sonico.com has more than 15 million users in Latin America.
- Friendster has approximately 60 million users, predominately in Asia, with just 17% in the US.
- ShoutBox, launched by bwin, is an example of a gambling specific social networking application. This app allows players to chat amongst themselves while playing casino games online and invite contacts to try games and participate in online tournaments (Bacot 2010).
- Betable, is a site where users can bet against family, friends and colleagues, and has been described as "Twitter for gambling" ('Betable' 2010).Individuals can nominate any type of bet and then share it through social media platforms including Facebook and Twitter. As an increasing number of players take up the bet, the pot grows and is spread between successful bettors, whilst the user that created the bet gets 30%. It is a form of betting exchange, but makes greater use of social media.

There are potentially strong opportunities to combine existing gambling products with social features; for example, IGS is developing a social networking application to be integrated into slot machines (Legato 2011). A "Friend Finder" will allow players to find a friend anywhere on the gaming floor and send them a text message. Similar applications could be integrated into online gambling platforms to heighten social interaction between players. Although the appropriate use of social networking and gaming continues to be a challenge for the online gambling industry, used correctly, these tools may allow operators to differentiate their products in a competitive market and provide greater customer engagement and enjoyment.

Mobile Gambling

Consumers are more and more comfortable using mobile phones for products and services such as mobile banking and ecommerce, and wireless Internet via 3G networks are increasingly available. The past few years have seen dramatic improvements to 3G technologies, greater availability of Wi-Fi, widespread use of powerful, reliable mobile devices with improved screens and an increase in the number of mobile applications that are commonly used and trusted.

The Pew Internet Project estimates that one in four US adults now uses mobile apps, and of those, nearly two in three people use their apps every day (Ezra 2011). The International Data Corporation ('Worldwide Smartphone Market' 2011) forecasts the global smartphone market to increase 55% year over year in 2011. Additional predictions suggest that by 2013, more people will access the Internet through mobile devices than through personal computers and that half of Americans will own and use smart phones by 2012. These are supported by reports that smart phone sales are now outselling personal computers, more than 350,000 Apple and 550,000 Android devices are activated daily and more than 15 billion apps have been downloaded by Apple users alone (Ezra 2011). Mobile phones and wireless devices are commonly used for social networking and information searches by customers of direct interest to online gambling operators. For example, research by Nielsen showed that out of 27,000 people surveyed in 55 countries, 21% planned to use mobile devices to obtain information about the 2010 FIFA World Cup and 9% would download an app to follow the action (Hearn 2010). This indicates the importance of online gambling operators engaging with sports fans and potential customers on mobile devices, given the preference for these by a growing number of individuals.

Online wagering sites were the first to take advantage of mobile phones and smart phones have evolved to have more screen space for operating systems (increasingly java-capable). These now show advanced graphics and allow programming and complicated displays required by online games (Owens 2010). Custom programs (apps) have also been developed for mobiles that enable almost all forms of online gambling to be conducted via mobile phones. Mobile betting allows gambling operators to interact with players in innovative ways, for example, enabling bettors to place bets at an event or while watching a game.

Estimates on the size of the mobile betting market vary widely. For many years now, the platform of mobile gambling has been heralded by the gambling industry as the 'next big thing' to revolutionise the nature of interactive gambling. In 2010, Juniper Research predicted that the total sum wagered on mobile casino games would pass US$48 billion by 2015. This prediction was based on high growth rates of mobile casinos, lotteries, and sports betting providers in major emerging markets and China, liberalisation of mobile gambling legislation in Europe, and the US modifying its policy of prohibition, so the figures are somewhat speculative. Results have fallen short of the bold predictions made a few years ago (iGaming Business 2011).

Factors that have inhibited the growth of mobile gambling include the lack of reliable and high quality networks, slow and small devices, difficulty in application availability and delivery as well as payment for customers, a lack of consumer confidence and regulatory restrictions (iGaming Business 2011; H2 Gambling Capital 2011). The lack of appropriate and easy payment methods remains a significant barrier to the growth of mobile gambling (iGaming Business 2011). In some jurisdictions, for example, the Netherlands, bets placed online can be added to mobile phone bills (Owens 2010), making payment simple, although in many cases separate accounts and payment systems are used. Similar developments in other jurisdictions would greatly aid the growth of the mobile gambling market. Key barriers to mobile gambling include regulatory hurdles and the ability to process payments. Vast improvements are required in the quantity and quality of payment solutions that allow customers to easily and quickly make deposits and withdrawals on mobile phones using their preferred method to allow massive expansion of this industry (iGaming Business 2011).

The global mobile gambling market was valued at US$2.8 billion in 2010, the vast majority of which was accounted for by mobile betting (GBGC 2011b; H2 Gambling Capital 2011). At the end of 2010 the mobile gambling market accounted for 9.8% of interactive and 0.6% of global gambling GGY (H2 Gambling Capital 2011). The mobile gambling market is forecast to grow to 12.9% and 0.9% respectively in 2011 and 2012 (H2 Gambling Capital 2011). Strong growth is predicted and the market is expected to reach US$5.3 billion by the end of 2015 (H2 Gambling Capital 2011).

Traditionally betting has made up the majority of the mobile gambling market at 76.74% of global GGY (H2 Gambling Capital 2011). However, in the next 5 years, product market share will shift towards gaming and lotteries as technology develops allowing players to use interactive software on mobile devices (H2 Gambling Capital 2011). In 2016 betting is predicted to account for 50.5% of the global mobile gambling market, with gaming, including bingo and slot machines accounting for 39.8% and lottery 9.7%. The increased popularity of live betting has been a positive development for mobile gambling given that up to 30% of bets on mobile are on live events (iGaming Business 2011). One example comes from William Hill, whose mobile betting now accounts for around 7% of its overall sportsbook revenues, due to a 600% growth in the first half of 2011 ('Mobile gambling to capture more of market' 2011). The online betting exchange Betfair has also reported that its investment in mobile betting, including mobile products in 17 different languages and a new iPad application, has been worthwhile (UK Press Association 2011). Betfair reported receiving 7.4 million bets placed on mobile devices in the 3 months to July 31, 2011, twice the number received during the same period in 2010.

There are currently a vast variety of free-play gambling apps available for smart phones. An analysis conducted in 2010 found 93 gambling apps for iPhones in addition to 250 poker apps, 42 sports betting apps, 393 casino apps and 49 slot apps (Korn et al. 2010). Real money gambling apps are also available for iPhones, however, these are subject to a lengthy application process. Since March 2011, Android has expressly prohibited the presence of any gambling application (iGaming Business 2011).

Given the substantial potential of the mobile gambling market in terms of growth and revenue, many online gambling operators, and land-based operators, are launching mobile apps. However, it is important for operators to do this in a systematic and considered manner to ensure that time and money spend developing and marketing apps is successful. Mobile apps may simply duplicate an online gambling site, however, mobile users typically want different features and mobile devices have different capabilities and strengths compared to computers (Ezra 2011). For example, apps should have large buttons that are easy to touch on screen and lots of clear space to enable easy navigation (Suggett 2011). Novelty apps include William Hill's 'Shake-a-Bet', which is intended for less serious players who can choose what they want to bet on, the amount that they want to bet, the number of selections and expected return and allows the app to suggest a random bet.

Apps may include interactive features that allow users to use a smartphone's camera, touch screen and include information in the real world. Such techniques may also integrate mobile gambling with marketing strategies, such as Betfair's recent deal with Britain's female beach volleyball team in which "quick response" codes are printed on player's bikini bottoms that individuals can register with smartphones to be taken to the website ('Bum future' 2011). Mobile apps must be constantly updated to ensure that they meet the demands of increasingly sophisticated devices and users, including their relevance with current topics and use of social media (Ezra 2011). There is tremendous capacity for mobile gambling and it is expected that many online gambling operators will move into this mode and provide increasingly sophisticated experiences for customers.

Conclusions

Abstract Substantially more research is required to understand Internet gambling and guide appropriate responses from policy makers and governments. In addition, educators, treatment providers and the community need to have a greater understanding of Internet gambling so that they may take appropriate actions in response to the risks posed by this form of gambling. Internet gambling offers many opportunities and challenges and has changed the nature of gambling at a global level. It is important that collaborative working partnerships be formed between researchers, industry operators, and policy makers to facilitate methodologically-sound empirical research that may accurately inform on the state of and impact of Internet gambling. Efforts must continue to ensure that this mode of gambling represents an entertainment activity with minimal risks and to mitigate the risks and challenges that accompany it.

Keywords Internet gambling • Online gaming • Regulation • Policy • Collaboration • Research • Trends • Overview • Future

Internet gambling is no longer a new phenomenon and mode of gambling, although there is still a relatively poor understanding of the use and impact of this activity. The dynamic nature of online gambling sites, evolving technology, innovative product offerings, and ever-shifting regulatory policies make it difficult to completely comprehend online gambling at a global level. The large number of sites and multitude of owners and operators spread across many international jurisdictions make it difficult to assemble a comprehensive picture of the online gambling field. Similarly, it is difficult to estimate the prevalence of Internet gambling within specific jurisdictions given the tendency for players to frequent multiple and offshore sites. Subsequently, it is difficult for politicians, governments, and regulators to enact appropriate policies due to the lack of information to guide these.

The increased trust and legitimacy of online gambling sites and willingness of players to bet online, coupled with the convenience and accessibility of online

S. Gainsbury, *Internet Gambling: Current Research Findings and Implications*,
SpringerBriefs in Behavioral Medicine 1, DOI 10.1007/978-1-4614-3390-3,
© Springer Science+Business Media, LLC 2012

gambling are all likely to be factors fostering participation in most international markets. Industry reports demonstrate a clear trend of increasing customer expenditure and associated revenue for online gambling, which includes computer-based and progressively more mobile gambling. Sustained growth is predicted as more jurisdictions legalise online gambling, technology continues to develop and the Internet becomes more accessible and existing land-based gambling and non-gambling companies move to enter this market. Politicians or policy makers that argue liberalising and regulating online gambling will introduce a new mode of gambling need to consider the extent of participation at illegal offshore sites as, despite attempts at prohibition, Internet gambling is highly accessible to any individual that has access to the Internet. Regulation will allow jurisdictions to demand high customer protection standards and increase the funds and taxes that remain within the jurisdiction. Despite uncertainties of the most effective strategies and regulations, it is now necessary to implement a cohesive framework to inform and shape a properly regulated Internet gambling environment.

What is clearly currently lacking in the field of Internet gambling is harmonization of regulations and policies between jurisdictions, including neighbouring jurisdictions, and even provinces or states within a single country. This is somewhat understandable as each jurisdiction needs to consider their own interests; however, the lack of consistency across the world creates substantial difficulties for players, who have difficulty understanding the best sites to play, operators, in abiding by different requirements, and policy makers due to the lack of uniform strategies on which to interpret impacts and subsequently base guidelines. Wider harmonization of regulatory frameworks would be based on the understanding that once an operator and online gambling site has been approved and demonstrated their propriety to conduct gambling, and agreed to the taxation requirements of relevant authorities, observance of common regulation would allow the operator to subsequently comply with requirements in other jurisdictions.

Harmonization of online gambling regulation would reduce the need of online gambling operators to spend substantial sums satisfying numerous licensing agreements and operating different sites for each jurisdiction. It would also have significant advantages for player protection and responsible gambling, as all participating jurisdictions could share relevant information for player identification and probity checks as well as a common self-exclusion list and even potentially player deposit and betting limits between operators. Consumers would benefit as online gambling sites are likely to be brought up to the highest common standards in order to meet requirements for licensing and those sites that are not regulated within the common understanding would be more obviously identified due to a single symbol designating the standards. Small efforts are being made in the direction of coordination and mutual agreements and it is hoped that these continue.

There have been increasing movements towards regulation of Internet gambling, arguably due to the futility of prohibition, the importance of providing a regulated environment, and economic incentives related to keeping gambling onshore. However, it may be irresponsible for governments to implement a new mode of gambling without fully understanding the potential impacts on individuals and communities. Academic research is increasingly examining Internet gambling, however, this research is still in its infancy, particularly in comparison to alcohol and tobacco research (European Commission 2011b). Concerns have been expressed about the potential social impacts of Internet gambling, particularly on youth and problem gamblers due to the ease of access of this mode of gambling. Numerous studies have reported higher rates of problem gambling in samples of Internet gamblers as compared to the general population and non-Internet gamblers. However, various methodological limitations constrain these results. Furthermore, it is uncertain whether Internet gamblers had existing problems related to other forms of gambling before gambling online, or whether the Internet leads to problems in those with no previous negative impacts.

The transition to Internet gambling from land-based or no gambling is an important area for research. The relationship between problem gambling and Internet gambling also needs consideration and it is important to conduct investigations of effective harm-minimisation policies and responsible gambling features that can be incorporated into online gambling sites. There is currently little evidence to guide the implementation of effective responsible gambling features, which are necessary to protect players from negative consequences. Due to player tracking and identification, it is possible that responsible gambling features and tools for online gambling sites may be highly effective and provide a safer playing environment than land-based venues. At the same time, due to highly competitive nature of the online gambling market, it is important for sites to provide customer protection strategies in an appealing manner that encourages players to use these rather than move to another site.

Further research is needed to understand how Internet gambling is being used in the context of other gambling behaviour and activities. Only preliminary results are available to guide the understanding of demographic characteristics of Internet gamblers and the motivations for using this mode of gambling. In particular, a conceptual model is needed, with supporting empirical evidence, to differentiate between subtypes of Internet gamblers and more fully explain the factors that initiate and motivate ongoing online gambling. Given the increased popularity and availability of Internet gambling, having a more complete understanding of the use of this activity is important to inform policy decisions. Such research is likely to require a multi-modal strategies including cooperation with gambling operators to access player databases and customers for surveys and focus groups, as well as prevalence surveys and other empirical methodologies.

To enable empirical studies, online gambling operators, governments, and researchers must work collaboratively to conduct valid and reliable research. Researchers should receive access to the large amounts of data collected by online gambling operators, after commercially sensitive information is removed, to enable analysis of gambling behaviour. This will have positive impacts on the industry by enabling greater customer understanding. Safe and responsible gambling represents a win-win solution for its clients and the industry. By satisfactorily ensuring that underage players are prohibited from playing, that responsible gambling solutions are in place, by ensuring honest, fair play and integrity, the regulatory processes and general population will be more likely to have a positive attitude toward Internet gaming. If properly regulated and responsible oversight is employed, the harms and risks to vulnerable populations may be minimized. The inclusion of responsible codes of conduct will help assure the public and will ultimately provide a safer product.

Gaps in Internet Gambling Research

- The relationship between online gambling and problem gambling
- What are the key risks and harms associated with online gambling?
- What policies and procedures can be implemented to protect vulnerable populations from Internet gambling-related harms?
- How can potential problem Internet gamblers be identified and what tools can be used to assist these players to gamble responsibly or cease gambling?
- What responsible gambling tools should be implemented to minimize harms and how can players be encouraged to use these?
- The relationship between youth and online gambling
- What are the key motivations, attractions and benefits of online gambling and do these differ amongst subgroups of players?
- How Internet gambling is used in relation to and in addition to other modes of gambling
- Do consumers use regulated onshore Internet sites if these are available and what motivates players to use offshore sites rather than regulated onshore sites?
- How will new technology impact online gambling and the manner in which individuals place bets online, what growth is expected for non-computer Internet gambling (e.g., mobile and interactive television)
- What international approaches to online gambling are most effective?

References

Abbott, M. (2007). Prospective problem gambling research: Contribution and potential. *International Gambling Studies, 7*, 123–144.

Abbott, M., Volberg, R., Bellringer, M., & Reith, G. (2004). A review of research on aspects of problem gambling. U.K. Responsibility in Gambling Trust

Alderney revokes Full Tilt Poker licences. (2011). *Gaming Intelligence.* Retrieved from http://gamingintelligence.com/business/13398-alderney-revokes-full-tilt-poker-licences

Allen Consulting Group. (2003). *Final report on issues related to Commonwealth interactive gambling regulation.* Retrieved from http://www.allenconsult.com.au/publications/download.php?id=286&type=pdf&file=1. Accessed 01 Sept 2010.

American Gaming Association. (2006). *2006 state of the states: The AGA survey of casino entertainment.* Washington, DC: American Gaming Association.

American Gaming Association. (2010). *2010 state of the states: The AGA survey of casino entertainment.* Washington, DC: American Gaming Association.

Anglican Diocese of Melbourne Social Responsibilities Committee. (2008). Submission to the *Senate Inquiry on the Poker Machine Harm Reduction Tax (Administration) Bill 2008.* Retrieved from www.aph.gov.au/senate/committee/clac_ctte/poker_machine_harm_reduct/submissions/sub08.pdf

Aristocrat secures first online deal with U.S casino. (2011). *Gaming Intelligence.* Retrieved from http://gamingintelligence.com/business/13445-aristocrat-secures-first-online-deal-with-us-casino

Atherton, M. (2006). The ultimate gamble. *The New Statesman.* Retrieved from http://www.newstatesman.com/200607240032. Accessed 6 Apr 2006.

Auriemma, T., & Lahey, W. (1999). *Gambling on the internet: Report to the international association of gaming regulators.* Paper presented at the 1999 IAGR conference, Paradise Island, The Bahamas.

Australian Associated Press. (2011). Younger Australians take up sports betting. *Herald Sun.* Retrieved from http://www.heraldsun.com.au/news/breaking-news/younger-australians-take-up-sports-betting/story-e6frf7jx-1226103086183

Australian National Institute for Public Policy. (2011). *Public opinion on gambling: ANU poll July 2011.* Canberra: Australian National University.

Bacot, J. (2010). Social networking and online casinos. *Ezine @rticles.* Retrieved from http://ezinearticles.com/?expert=Jason_Bacot&q=Social+Networking+and+Online+Casinos

Bad debts rise for e-gaming firms. (2011). *Global Betting & Gaming Consultancy.* Retrieved from http://www.gbgc.com/2010/04/bad-debts-rise-for-e-gaming-firms/

Balding, R. (2011). Some European countries so no to online gambling. *Casino Advisor.* Retrieved from http://www.casinoadvisor.com/some-european-countries-say-no-to-online-gambling-news-item.html

Balfour, F. (2011). Betting sites challenge venerable Hong Kong track. *Bloomberg Businessweek*. Retrieved from http://articles.sfgate.com/2011-02-22/business/28617562_1_pool-bets-online-bookmakers-hong-kong-jockey-club

Barker, J. (2007). *Owning a sportsbook is not a licence to print money*. Retrieved from http://www.puntingace.com/bettingguide/own_sportsbook.html

Basham, P., & White, K. (2002). *Gambling with our future? The costs and benefits of legalised gambling*. Vancouver: Fraser Institute.

BC Partnership for Responsible Gambling. (2011). *Internet Gambling*. Retrieved from http://www.bcresponsiblegambling.ca/other/internet.html

Beach, S. (2009). China jails 20 in 'Biggest-ever' internet gambling case: Report. *China Digital Times*. Retrieved from http://chinadigitaltimes.net/2009/02/china-jails-20-in-biggest-ever-internet-gambling-case-report/

Bennett, J. (2011a). Betfair Australia CEO to leave in February. *EGaming Review Magazine*. Retrieved from http://www.egrmagazine.com/news/1694492/betfair-australia-ceo-to-leave-in-february.thtml?utm_source=daily-snapshot&utm_medium=newsletter&utm_campaign=daily-snapshot. 15 Sept 2011.

Bennett, J. (2011b). EC raises doubts over German gambling law. *EGaming Review Magazine*. Retrieved from http://www.egrmagazine.com/news/1679957/ec-raises-doubts-over-german-gambling-law.thtml?utm_source=daily-snapshot&utm_medium=newsletter&utm_campaign=daily-snapshot

Bennett, J. (2011c). An industry awaits Part 4 – monetisation of social media. *EGaming Review Magazine*. Retrieved from http://www.egrmagazine.com/features/870907/2011-an-industry-awaits-part-4-monetisation-of-social-media.thtml

Benston, L. (2010). Question evolving from legalization debate: How to tax online casinos? *Las Vegas Sun*. Retrieved from http://www.lasvegassun.com/news/2010/may/24/how-tax-online-casinos/

Bernhard, B. J., Lucas, A. F., & Shampaner, E. (2007). *Internet gambling in Nevada*. Las Vegas: International Gaming Institute/University of Nevada.

Berzon, A. (2011). MGM resorts to state online game to woo new customers. *The Wall Street Journal*. Retrieved from http://online.wsj.com/article/SB1000142405297020347680457661373218235846 2.html?mod=dist_smartbrief

Betable: Social media betting. (2010). *MoneyWatch*. Retrieved from http://money-watch.co.uk/7264/betable-social-media-betting

Betfair kept massive car data theft quiet. (2011). *Finextra*. Retrieved from http://www.finextra.com/news/fullstory.aspx?newsitemid=23022

Bjerg, O. (2010). Problem gambling in poker: Money, rationality and control in a skill-based social game. *International Gambling Studies, 10*, 239–254.

Blaszczynski, A., Ladouceur, R., & Shaffer, H. (2004). A science-based framework for responsible gambling: The Reno model. *Journal of Gambling Studies, 20*, 301–317.

Blaszczynski, A., Ladouceur, R., Nower, L., & Shaffer, H. (2005). *Informed choice and gambling: Principles for consumer protection*. Melbourne: Australian Gaming Council.

Bonke, J. (2007). *Ludomani i Danmark II Faktorer af betydning for spilleproblemer [Gambling in Denmark II Factors involved in problem gambling]* (Rep. No. 07:14). Copenhagen: Institute of Social Research

Braverman, J., & Shaffer, H. J. (2010). How do gamblers start gambling: Identifying behavioural markers for high-risk internet gambling. *European Journal of Public Health*. doi:10.1093/eurpub/ckp232.

Breen, H., & Zimmerman, M. (2002). Rapid onset of pathological gambling in machine gamblers. *Journal of Gambling Studies, 18*, 31–43.

Breen, H., Buultjens, J., & Hing, N. (2005). Evaluating implementation of a voluntary responsible gambling code in Queensland, Australia. *International Journal of Mental Health and Addiction, 3*, 15–25.

Broda, A., LaPlante, D., Nelson, A., LaBrie, R., Bosworth, L., & Shaffer, H. (2008). Virtual harm reduction efforts for internet gambling: Effects of deposit limits on actual internet sports gambling behaviour. *Harm Reduction Journal, 5*, 5–27.

Brunker, M. (2011). Indicted poker websites bound for bankruptcy: Collapse of Absolute Poker and UB sites mean U.S. players may lost deposits. *MSNBC*. Retrieved from http://www.msnbc.msn.com/id/42906061/ns/business-us_business/

Bum future for women's beach volleyball: Is this the tackiest sports ad deal? (2011). *News.com.au*. Retrieved from http://www.news.com.au/business/bum-future-for-volleyball-is-this-the-tackiest-sport-ad-deal/story-e6frfm1i-1226111440011

Bundeszentrale für gesundheitliche Aufklärung. (2010). *Glücksspielverhalten in Deutchland 2007 und 2009: Ergebnisse aus zwei represäntativen bevölkerungsbefragnungen*. Köln, Bundeszentrale für gesundheitliche Aufklärung: 81.

Camelot. (2011). Camelot sets new National Lottery sales record. *Press Release*. Retrieved from http://www.camelotgroup.co.uk/news/corporate/CamelotsetsnewNationalLotterysalesrecord030611

Canadian Press (2011). Ontario bets big on online gambling. *The Globe and Mail*. Retrieved from http://www.theglobeandmail.com/news/national/ontario/ontario-bets-big-on-online-gambling/article1668179/

Capone, A. (2009). The meaningless sanction: The World Trade Organization's inability to control its larger members and failure to help its smaller members. *Selected Words of Andrew Capone*. Retrieved from http://works.bepress.com/andrew_capone/1

Carpenter, M. (2005). More women betting on online poker. Pittsburgh Post Gazette.

Carr, J. (2011). Keeping children safe online. *EGBA News, 9*, 3.

Casino City Online. (2011). http://online.casinocity.com/. Accessed 23 July 2011.

Cass. (2011). Alderney as a gambling jurisdiction shines. *Online Casino News*. Retrieved from http://www.cassaon-casino.com/blog/online-casino-news/alderney-as-a-gambling-jurisdiction-shines

Catania, F. (2011). Pressing mute? *Global Gaming Business Magazine, 10* (10).

CEN Workshop. (2010). *Draft CEN Workshop agreement: Responsible remote gambling measures*. Retrieved from http://www.cen.eu/cen/Sectors/TechnicalCommitteesWorkshops/Workshops/Pages/WS58eGambling.aspx

Centre for the Digital Future. (2008). *World Internet Project: International Report 2008*. Retrieved from http://www.digitalcenter.org/pages/site_content.asp?intGlobalId=42

Chaivarlis, E. (2011). Chad Elie and John Campos released. *POKERnews Global*. Retrieved from http://www.pokernews.com/news/2011/04/chad-elie-and-john-campos-released-10243.htm

Charif, M. (2011). Show me the money: Social games, virtual currency and gambling. *iGaming Business*. Retrieved from http://www.harrishagan.com/publications/

Chee, F. Y. (2011). Top EU court backs gambling monopolies. *Reuters US Edition*. Retrieved from http://www.reuters.com/article/2011/09/15/court-austria-gambling-idUSLDE78E0B420110915

Chen, Z. (2005). Towards online shopping in New Zealand. *Journal of Electronic Commerce Research*. Retrieved from http://www.allbusiness.com/buying_exiting_businesses/3504614-1.html

Christiansen Capital Advisors. (2005). *eGaming Data Report*. Retrieved from http://www.cca-i.com/primary%20navigation/online%20data%20store/internet_gambling_data.htm

Christiansen Capital Advisors. (2007). Global internet gambling revenue estimates and projections (2001–2010). Retrieved from http://www.ccai.com/Primary%20Navigation/Online%20Data%20Store/internet_gambling_dat.hem

Church-Sanders, R. (2010). *The global business of online casinos: Outlook, forecasts and analysis*. London: iGaming Business.

Church-Sanders, R. (2011). *Online sports betting: A market assessment and outlook*. London: iGaming Business.

Coltman, T., Devinney, T., Latekefu, A., & Midgley, D. (2001). E-business: Revolution, evolution, or hype? *California Management Review, 44*, 57–86.

Commission, E. (2011). *Green paper on on-line gambling in the internal market*. Brussels: European Commission.

Constine, J. (2011). Facebook's ad guidelines now permit offline gambling, lotteries and dietary supplements. *Inside Facebook*. Retrieved from http://www.insidefacebook.com/2011/08/24/ad-guidelines-gambling-lotteries-dietary-supplements/

Corney, R., & Davis, J. (2010). The attractions and risks of internet gambling for women: A qualitative study. *Journal of Gambling Issues, 24*, 121–139.

Cotte, J., & Latour, K. (2009). Blackjack in the kitchen: Understanding online versus casino gambling. *Journal of Consumer Research, 35*, 742–758.

Credit cards 'have vague interest rates'. (2011). *UK Net Guide*. Retrieved from http://www.uknet guide.co.uk/Latest-News/Credit-cards-have-vague-interest-rates-800736942.html

Crumb, M. (2010). Cash-strapped states of all in on gambling. *Associated Press*. Retrieved from http://www.msnbc.msn.com/id/35879023/ns/us_news-life/t/cash-strapped-states-go-all-gambling/

Cunningham, J. A., Sdao-Jarvie, K., Koski-Jännes, A., & Breslin, F. C. (2001). Motivating change at assessment for alcohol treatment. *Journal of Substance Abuse Treatment, 20*, 301–304.

Cunningham, J. A., Hodgins, D. C., Toneatto, T., Rai, A., & Cordingley, J. (2009). Pilot study of personalized feedback intervention for problem gamblers. *Behavior Therapy, 40*, 219–224.

Defence in NYC prosecution says online poker isn't gambling, it's a game of skill. (2011). *Washington Post*. Retrieved from http://www.washingtonpost.com/business/technology/defense-in-nyc-prosecution-says-online-poker-isnt-gambling-its-a-game-of-skill/2011/10/03/gIQAVpGnIL_story.html

Delfabbro, P. (2008). *Australasian gambling review* (3rd ed.). Adelaide: Independent Gambling Authority of South Australia.

Delfabbro, P., Lahn, J., & Grabosky, P. (2005). *Adolescent gambling in the ACT*. Canberra: Centre for Gambling Research, Australian National University.

Department for Culture, Media and Sport, Gambling Act. (2005). Retrieved from http://www.culture.gov.uk/what_we_do/gambling_and_racing/3305.aspx

Department for Social Development. (2010). Northern Ireland gambling prevalence survey 2010. Belfast: Department for Social Development.

Department of Broadband Communications and the Digital Economy. (2011). *Review of the interactive gambling act 2011: Call for submissions*. Canberra: Department of Broadband Communications and the Digital Economy.

Derevensky, J. (2008). Gambling behaviors and adolescent substance abuse disorders. In Y. Kaminer & O. G. Buckstein (Eds.), *Adolescent substance abuse: Psychiatric comorbidity and high risk behaviors* (pp. 399–429). New York: Haworth.

Derevensky, J. (2009). *Internet gambling among youth: Cause for concern!* National Council on Problem Gambling Conference, Singapore.

Derevensky, J., & Gupta, R. (2002). Youth gambling: A clinical and research perspective. *The Electronic Journal of Gambling Issues, 2*. http://www.camh.net/egambling/issue2/feature/ Accessed 28 Jan 2008.

Derevensky, J. L., & Gupta, R. (2007). Internet gambling amongst adolescents: A growing concern. *International Journal of Mental Health and Addictions, 5*, 93–101.

Derevensky, J., Sklar, A., Gupta, R., Messerlian, C., Laroche, M., & Mansour, S. (2007). *The effects of gambling advertisements on child and adolescent gambling attitudes and behaviors (Les effets de la publicité sur les attitudes et les comportements de jeu des enfants et des adolescents)*. Report prepared for the Fonds de recherché en santé du Québec (FRSQ), Québec.

Derevensky, J., Sklar, A., Gupta, R., & Messerlian, C. (2010). An empirical study examining the impact of gambling advertisements on adolescent gambling attitudes and behaviours. *International Journal of Mental Health and Addiction, 8*, 21–34.

Dinev, T., Bellotto, M., Hart, P., Russo, V., Serra, I., & Colautti, C. (2006). Privacy calculus model in e-commerce: A study of Italy and the United States. *European Journal of Information Systems, 15*, 389–402.

DoJ attack leaves UB and Absolute Poker bankrupt. (2011). *Poker News Report*. Retrieved from http://www.pokernewsreport.com/doj-attack-leaves-ub-and-absolute-poker-bankrupt-2068

DoJ brings more charges against Full Tilt. (2011). *Gaming Intelligence*. Retrieved from http://www.gamingintelligence.com/business/13310-doj-brings-more-charges-against-full-tilt

Donoghue, A., & Healy, H. (2011). The changing face of gaming. *EGaming Review Magazine.* Retrieved from http://www.egrmagazine.com/blog/1696682/the-changing-face-of-gaming. thtml?utm_source=daily-snapshot&utm_medium=newsletter&utm_campaign=daily-snapshot

Dowling, N., Jackson, A., Thomas, S., & Frydenberg, E. (2010). *Children at risk of developing problem gambling.* Melbourne: The Problem Gambling Research and Treatment Centre.

Doyle, J. (2008). Cross cultural communication – Can you meet the challenge? *Casino & Gaming International, 2,* 41–44.

Dragicevic, S. (2011). Time for change: The industry's approach to self-exclusion. *World Online Gambling Law Report, 10*(7), 6–8.

Dragicevic, S., Tsogas, G., & Kudic, A. (2011). Analysis of casino online gambling data in relation to behavioural risk markers for high-risk gambling and player protection. *International Gambling Studies, 11,* 377–391.

Eadington, W. R. (1995). Economic development and the introduction of casinos: Myths and realities. *Economic Development Review, Fall,* 51–54

Eadington, W. R. (2004). The future of online gambling in the United States and elsewhere. *Journal of Public Policy & Marketing, 23,* 214–219.

eCOGRA. (2007). *An exploratory investigation in the attitudes and behaviours of internet Casino and poker players.* Nottingham: Institute for the study of gambling and commercial gaming: Nottingham Trent University.

Edwards, S., Li, H., & Lee, J. (2002). Forced exposure and psychological reactance: Antecedents and consequences of the perceived intrusiveness of pop-up ads. *Journal of Advertising, 31,* 83–95.

Eldon, E. (2011). Zynga hires team from poker industry service provider MarketZero. *Inside Social Games.* Retrieved from http://www.insidesocialgames.com/2011/04/05/zynga-hires-team-from-poker-industry-service-provider-marketzero/

European Parliament (2008). *Online gambling: Focusing on integrity and a code of conduct for gambling.* European Parliament, Policy Department, Economic and Scientific Policy, IP/A/IMCO/FWC/2006-186/C1/SC2.

European Commission (2011a). *Green paper on on-line gambling in the Internal Market.* Brussels: European Commission.

European Commission. (2011b). *Conclusions: Workshop on online gambling: Detection and prevention of problem gambling and gambling addiction.* Brussels. Retrieved from http://ec.europa.eu/internal_market/services/docs/gambling/workshops/workshop-ii-conclusions_en.pdf

European Commission. (2011c). *Conclusions: Workshop on online gambling: Prevention of fraud and money laundering.* Brussels. Retrieved from http://ec.europa.eu/internal_market/services/docs/gambling/workshops/workshop-iv-conclusions_en.pdf

European Committee for Standardization. (2011). *Responsible remote gambling measures: CEN Workshop agreement.* Brussels: CEN-CENELEC Management Centre.

European Gaming and Betting Association. (2011). *Written submission to the green paper on online gambling in the internal market.* Brussels: European Gaming and Betting Association.

Europeans take a gamble online. (2002). *NetValue survey.* Retrieved from http://www.nua.ie/surveys/analysis/weekly_editorial/archives/issue1no307.html

Ezra, A. (2011). Casinos going mobile. *Gaming Business, 10*(9). Accessed from http://ggbmagazine.com/issue/vol-10-no-9-september-2011/article/casinos-going-mobile

Fall in disputes resolved in favour of players, says eCOGRA. (2011) *Gaming intelligence.* Retrieved from http://www.gamingintelligence.com/legal/12621-fall-in-disputes-resolved-in-favour-of-players-says-ecogra

Fang Y., Qureshi I., McCole P., & Ramsey, E. (2007). The moderating role of perceived effectiveness of third party control on trust and online repurchasing intentions. *Proceedings, Americas conference on information systems,* pp. 1–18.

Felsher, J., Derevensky, J., & Gupta, R. (2004). Lottery playing amongst youth: Implications for prevention and social policy. *Journal of Gambling Studies, 20,* 127–153.

Fiedler, I. C., & Rock, J. P. (2009). Quantifying skill in games: Theory and empirical evidence for poker. *Gaming Law Review & Economics, 13*(1), 50–57.

Financial Action Task Force. (2001) *FATF-XII: Report on money laundering typologies (2000-2001)*.

Flood, K. (2011). How land based casinos can leverage social networks and social games to improve their business. *Kevin's Corner*. Retrieved from http://kevinflood.blogspot.com/2011/05/significance-of-harrahs-playtika.html

Focal Research Consultants. (2008). *2007 Nova Scotia adult gambling prevalence study*. Nova Scotia Department of Health Promotion and Protection. Retrieved from http://www.gov.ns.ca/ohp/publications/Adult_Gambling_Report.pdf

Form S-I Registration Statement. (2011). *U.S. Securities and Exchange Commission* Website.

Gaboury, A., & Ladouceur, R. (1989). Erroneous perceptions and gambling. *Journal of Social Behavior and Personality, 4*, 411–420.

Gainsbury, S. (2010). Response to the productivity commission inquiry into gambling: Online gaming and the interactive gambling act. *Gambling Research, 22*(2), 3–12.

Gainsbury, S. (2011). Player account-based gambling: Potentials for behaviour-based research methodologies. *International Gambling Studies, 11*(2), 153–171.

Gainsbury, S., & Blaszczynski, A. (2011a). Online self-guided interventions for the treatment of problem gambling. *International Gambling Studies, 11*, 289–308.

Gainsbury, S., & Blaszczynski, A. (2011b). *Invited submission to the joint select committee on gambling reform inquiry into interactive gambling*. Retrieved from http://www.aph.gov.au/senate/committee/gamblingreform_ctte/interactive_online_gambling_advertising/submissions.htm

Gainsbury, S., & Wood, R. (2011). Internet gambling policy in critical comparative perspective: The effectiveness of existing regulatory frameworks. *International Gambling Studies, 11*, 309–323.

Gainsbury, S., Parke, J., & Suhonen, N. (2011). *Consumer attitudes towards Internet gambling: Player perceptions of consumer protection, responsible gambling policies and regulation of online gambling sites*. Manuscript submitted for publication.

Gambling Commission. (2008). *What to look out for when gambling online*. Retrieved from http://www.gamblingcommission.gov.uk/up/oaddocs/publications/document/online%20gambling.pdf. Accessed 30 Nov 2008.

Gambling commission prevalence survey flawed. (2011). *Global betting & gaming consultants*. Retrieved from http://www.gbgc.com/2011/02/

Games and Casino (2006). *Blacklisted casinos*. Retrieved from http://www.gamesandcasino.com/blacklist.htm

Gaming Zion (2011). *UK watchdog bans contentious gambling ad*. Retrieved from http://gaming-zion.com/gamblingnews/uk-watchdog-bans-contentious-gambling-ad-1176

Glasser, A. J. (2011).The Top 25 Facebook Games For September 2011. Inside Social Games.

Global Betting and Gaming Consultants. (2010). Global Gaming Report (5th ed.). Castletown, Isle of Man, British Isles: Author

Global Betting and Gaming Consultants. (2011a). Global gaming report (6th ed.). Castletown/Isle of Man/British Isles: Author

Global Betting & Gaming Consultants. (2011b). Mobile gambling report 2011. Isle of Man/British Isles: Global Betting & Gaming Consultants.

Gold Media. (2010). *Germany football fans resort to foreign-based sports betting services*. Berlin: Gold Media. Retrieved from http://www.goldmedia.com/en/press/newsroom/study-betting-and-gambling-in-germany.html?PHPSESSID=b2b364d590ab42b70004ca93f22a8c71#c7036

Goodley, S. (2011). Newly merged Bwin.party rocked by German betting tax proposals. *Guardian.co.uk*. Retrieved from http://www.guardian.co.uk/business/2011/apr/06/bwin-party-rocked-by-german-betting-tax

Gray, R. (2011). *New Zealanders'participation in gambling. Results from the 2010 health and lifestyle survey*. Wellington: Health Sponsorship Council.

Griffiths, M. D. (2001). Internet gambling: Preliminary results of the first UK prevalence study. eGambling: *The Electronic Journal of Gambling Issues*. Retrieved from http://www.camh.net/egambling/issue5/research/griffiths_article.html

Griffiths, M. (2003). Internet gambling: Issues, concerns, and recommendations. *Cyberpsychology & Behavior, 6*(6), 557–568.

Griffiths, M. (2006). Is internet gambling more addictive than casino gambling. *Casino and Gaming International, 2,* 85–91.

Griffiths, M. D., & Barnes, A. (2008). Internet gambling: An online empirical study among student gamblers. *International Journal of Mental Health and Addiction, 6,* 194–204.

Griffiths, M. D., & Parke, J. (2002). The social impact of internet gambling. *Social Science Computer Review, 20,* 312–320.

Griffiths, M., & Wood, R. T. A. (2000). Risk factors in adolescence: The case of gambling, videogame playing, and the internet. *Journal of Gambling Studies, 16,* 199–225.

Griffiths, M., Wardle, H., Orford, J., Sproston, K., & Erens, B. (2009a). Sociodemographic correlates of internet gambling: Findings from the 2007 British gambling prevalence survey. *Cyberpsychology & Behavior, 12,* 199–202.

Griffiths, M. D., Wood, R. T. A., & Parke, J. (2009b). Social responsibility tools in online gambling: A survey of attitudes and behavior among internet gamblers. *Cyberpsychology & Behavior, 12,* 413–421.

Grinols, E. L. (2001). Cutting the cards and craps: Right thinking about gambling economics. Retrieved from http://www.voicesoftheheartland.org/Reference/Grinols-Cutting%20Cards%20and%20Craps.pdf]

Grohman, C. (2006). Reconsidering regulation: A historical view of the legality of internet poker and discussion of the internet gambling ban of 2006. *Journal of Legal Technology Risk Management, 1,* 34–74.

Gros, R. (2011a). Up against the wall. *Global Gaming Business, 10*(7).

Gros, R. (2011b). Moment of truth. *Global Gaming Business, 10*(10).

Grun, L., & McKeigue, P. (2000). Prevalence of excessive gambling before and after the introduction of a national lottery in the United Kingdom: Another example of the single distribution theory. *Addiction, 95,* 959–966.

Guo, L., Xiao, J. J., & Tang, C. (2009). Understanding the psychological process underlying customer satisfaction and retention in a relational service. *Journal of Business Research, 62,* 1152–1159.

H2 Gambling Capital. (2011). *Gambling goes mobile.* London: H2 Gambling Capital.

Haefeli, J., Lischer, S., & Schwarx, J. (2011). Early detection items and responsible gambling features for online gambling. *International Gambling Studies, 11,* 273–288.

Hammer, R. (2001). Does internet gambling strengthen the US economy? Don't bet on it. *Federal Communications Law Journal, 54,* 103–128.

Hayer, T., & Meyer, G. (2011). Internet self-exclusion: Characteristics of self-excluded gamblers and preliminary evidence for its effectiveness. *International Journal of Mental Health & Addictions, 9,* 296–307.

Hearn, L. (2010). Football fans flock to small screen. Football fans flock to small screen. *Sydney Morning Herald.* Retrieved from http://www.smh.com.au/digital-life/mobiles/football-fans-flock-to-small-screen-20100609-xvs2.html

Hennessry, N. (2011). Online gambling harms mortgage applications. *Irish Examiner.com.* Retrieved from http://www.irishexaminer.com/ireland/online-gambling-harms-mortgage-applications-166507.html#ixzz1X77WIKAq

Henwood, D. (2011). *Sports betting: The big picture.* EGR Live, Business Design Centre, London. Retrieved from http://www.h2gc.com/news.php?article=H2+Gambling+Capital+Presentations+-+EGR+Live+May+2011

Hing, N. (2004). *The efficacy of responsible gambling measures in NSW clubs: The gamblers' perspective.* Australian Gaming Council. Retrieved from http://www.austgamingcouncil.org.au/images/pdf/eLibrary/2755.pdf

Holliday, S. (2010). *Global interactive gambling universe: H2 market forecast/sector update.* H2 Gambling Capital. Retrieved from http://www.h2gc.com/news.php?article=H2+Gambling+Ca pital+Presentations+May+2010

Holliday, S. (2011). *The balance of power in global eGaming.* EGR Live, Business Design Centre, London. Retrieved from http://www.h2gc.com/news.php?article=H2+Gambling+Capital+Pres entations+-+EGR+Live+May+2011

Holtgrave, T. (2009). Gambling, gambling activities, and problem gambling. *Psychology of Addictive Behaviors, 23,* 295–302.

Hopley, A. A. B., & Nicki, R. M. (2010). Predictive factors of excessive online poker playing. *Cyberpsychology, Behaviour & Social Networking, 12,* 379–385.

Hornbuckle, W. (2003). Testimony to the House Judiciary Committee on Crime, Terrorism, and Homeland Security. Retrieved from http://www.house.gov

Iceland, S. (2006). *Statistical series: Information technology.* Reykjavík: Author.

iGaming Business. (2009). *The global business of poker report* (3rd ed.). London: iGaming Business.

iGaming Business. (2011). *Mobile gambling report: Opportunities for the industry.* London: iGaming Business.

Ihaka, J. (2011). Sports punters cheated of $900,000. *NZHerald.co.nz.* Retrieved from http://www. nzherald.co.nz/nz/news/article.cfm?c_id=1&objectid=10755395

Independent Sport Panel. (2009). The future of sport in Australia Retrieved from http://www. sportpanel.org.au/internet/sportpanel/publishing.nsf/Content/crawford-report-full

India and Asia new ground for online casino operators. (2011). *Online-Casinos.com.* Retrieved from http://www.online-casinos.com/news/news1710818.asp

Internal Market and Consumer Protection Committee. (2011). Press release. Stronger cooperation needed on online gambling, MEPs say. *European Parliament.* Retrieved from http://www. europarl.europa.eu/en/pressroom/content/20111003IPR28106/html/Stronger-cooperation-needed-on-online-gambling-MEPs-say

Ipsos Reid. (2005). *Online poker in North America: A syndicated study.* Retrieved from http:// www.ipsos-na.com

Ipsos Reid. (2010). Internet gambling in Canada: Public perception and behaviour. *2010 Canadian Gaming Summit, Canadian Gaming Association.* Retrieved from http://www.canadiangaming. ca/industry-facts/cga-research-a-studies/62-internet-gaming-in-canada-public-perception-and-behaviour.html

Jackson, S. (2008). Internet lottery: Reaching out to an untapped segment. *Lottery Insights,* 20–21

Jackson, A., Dowling, N., Thomas, S., Bond, L., & Patton, G. (2008). Adolescent gambling behaviour and attitudes: A prevalence study and correlates in an Australian population. *International Journal of Mental Health and Addiction, 6,* 325–352.

Jawad, C., & Griffiths, S. (2008). *A critical analysis of online gambling websites.* 2008 EBEN-UK annual conference, Cambridge.

Jiménez-Murcia, S., Stinchfield, R., Fernández-Aranda, F., Santamaría, J., Granero, R., Penelo, E., Menchon, J. et al. (2011). Are online pathological gamblers different from non-online Pathological Gamblers on demographics, gambling problem severity, psychopathology, and personality characteristics? *International Gambling Studies, 11,* 325–337.

Johan, A. (2011). UK Gambling Commission releases new statistics. *Gambling Kingz.* Retrieved from http://www.gamblingkingz.com/news/2011/08/02/uk-gambling-commission-releases-new-statistics.asp

Johnson, C., & Hult, P. (2008). *Web buyers and their expectations grow up: Experienced web buyers are becoming the new mainstream.* Cambridge: Forrest Research.

Jolley, B., Mizerski, R., & Olaru, D. (2006). How habit and satisfaction affects player retention for online gambling. *Journal of Business Research, 59,* 770–777.

Jonsson, J. (2008) *Responsible gaming and gambling problems among 3000 Swedish internet poker players.* 7th European association for the study of gambling conference. Retrieved from http://www.assissa.eu/easg/thursday/1400-ses3/jonsson_jakob.pdf

Juniper Research. (2010). *Mobile gambling wagers to surpass $48bn by 2015.* Press release. Retrieved from http://www.juniperresearch.com/viewpressrelease.php?pr=204

Kelleher, G. (2010). *The interactive gambling industry: Key trends 2010.* Prague: iGaming Supershow.

Kelly, J. (2008). A tale of two jurisdictions: US and Canada. *Casino & Gaming International, 3,* 17–21.

Kelly, J. M., Dhar, Z., & Verbiest, T. (2007). Poker and the law: Is it a game of skill or chance and legally does it matter? *Gaming Law Review, 11,* 190–202.

Kim, E. (2008). Survey shows free online gambling puts teens at risk; perceived as safe, it can groom youths for wager activities. *Statesman Journal.* Retrieved from http://www.responsible gambling.org/articles/082908_35.pdf

Kimber, G. (2011). Player protection, the final frontier. *eGaming Review,* Retrieved from: http://www.egrmagazine.com/blog/1682447/player-protection-the-final-frontier.thtml

Kingsley, R. (2011). Garman State passes online gambling legislation. *Casino Advisor.* Retrieved from http://www.responsiblegambling.org/staffsearch/latest_news_articles_details.cfm?intID= 13173

Koning, R., & van Velzen, B. (2009). Betting exchanges: The future of sports betting? *International Journal of Sport Finance, 4,* 42–62.

Korn, D. (2005). *Commercial gambling advertising: Possible impact on youth knowledge, attitudes, beliefs and behavioural intentions.* Guelph: Ontario Problem Gambling Research Centre.

Korn, D., Norman, C., & Reynolds, J. (2010). *Youth, gambling and Web 2.0: Towards and understanding of the net generation and how they gamble.* Guelph: Ontario Problem Gambling Research Centre.

KPMG International. (2010). Online gaming: A gamble or a sure bet? Author.

Krafcik, C. (2011). *US internet lobbying spend H1.* Washington, DC: Gambling Compliance.

Kun, B., Balazs, H., Arnold, P., Paksi, B., & Demetrovics, Z. (2011). Gambling in Western and Eastern Europe: The example of Hungary. *Journal of Gambling Studies.* doi:10.1007/s10899-011-9242-4.

LaBrie, R. A., Kaplan, S. A., Laplante, D. A., Nelson, S. E., & Shaffer, H. J. (2008). Inside the virtual casino: A prospective longitudinal study of actual Internet casino gambling. *European Journal of Public Health, 18,* 410–416.

LaBrie, R., LaPlante, D., Nelson, S., Schumann, A., & Shaffer, H. (2007). Assessing the playing field: A prospective longitudinal study of internet sports gambling behavior. *Journal of Gambling Studies, 23,* 347–362.

Ladd, G., & Petry, N. (2002). Disordered gambling among university-based medical and dental patients: A focus on internet gambling. *Psychology of Addictive Behaviors, 16,* 76–79.

Ladouceur, R., Sylvain, C., Boutin, C., Lachance, S., Doucet, C., Leblond, J., et al. (2001). Cognitive treatment of pathological gambling. *The Journal of Nervous and Mental Disease, 189,* 774–780.

Lamont, M., Hing, N., & Gainsbury, S. (2011). Gambling on sport sponsorship: A conceptual framework for research and regulatory review. *Sport Management Review, 14,* 246–257.

LaPlante, D., & Shaffer, H. (2007). Understanding the influence of gambling opportunities: Expanding exposure models to include adaptation'. *The American Journal of Orthopsychiatry, 77,* 616–623.

LaPlante, D., Schumann, A., LaBrie, R., & Shaffer, H. (2008). Population trends in internet sports gambling. *Computers in Human Behavior, 24,* 2399–2414.

LaPlante, D. A., Nelson, S. E., LaBrie, R. A., & Shaffer, H. J. (2009). The relationships between disordered gambling, type of gambling, and gambling involvement in the British Gambling Prevalence Survey 2007. *European Journal of Public Health Advance online publication.* doi:10.1093/eurpub/ckp177.

Legato, F. (2011). R&D power: International game technology. *Global Gaming Business Magazine, 10*(10).

Levine, M. (2010). *Current and future trends driving Australia's gambling sector.* Sydney: Gambling Reform Summit.

Lipton, M. D., & Weber, K. J. (2005). *The legality of internet gambling in Canada*. Toronto: Elkind, Lipton, & Jacobs. Retrieved from https://dspace.ucalgary.ca/bitstream/1880/47421/4/lipton.pdf

Lloyd, J., Doll, H., Hawton, K., Dutton, W. H., Geddes, J. R., Goodwin, G. M., & Rogers, R. D. (2010). Internet gamblers: A latent class analysis of their behaviours and health experiences. *Journal of Gambling Studies, 26*, 387–399.

MacKay, T.-L. (2005). *Betting on youth: Adolescent internet gambling in Canada*. Discovery, Niagara Falls, ON. Retrieved from http://www.responsiblegambling.org/articles/Terri_Lynn_MacKay_discovery_2005.pdf

Mangion, G. (2010). Perspective from Malta: Money laundering and its relation to online gambling. *Gaming Law Review & Economics, 14*(5), 363–370.

Marrison, J. (2011). E-Gaming companies making presence felt in Argentina. *Global Betting & Gaming Consultants*. Retrieved from http://www.gbgc.com/2011/03/e-gaming-companies-making-presence-felt-in-argentina/

McBride, J. (2006). Internet gambling among youth: A preliminary examination. *International Centre for Youth Gambling Problems & High-Risk Behaviors Newsletter, 6*, 1.

McBride, J., & Derevensky, J. (2009). Internet gambling behaviour in a sample of online gamblers. *International Journal of Mental Health and Addiction, 7*, 149–167.

McCole, P., Ramsey, E., & Williams, J. (2010). Trust considerations on attitudes towards online purchasing: The moderating effect of privacy and security concerns. *Journal of Business Research, 63*, 1018–1024.

McCormack, A., & Griffiths, M. (2010). Motivating and inhibiting factors in online gambling behaviour: A grounded theory study. *International Journal of Mental Health and Addiction*. doi:Advance online publication DOI: 10.1007/s11469-010-9300-7.

McCormack, A., & Griffiths, M. (2011). What differentiates professional poker players from recreational poker players? A qualitative interview study. *International Journal of Mental Health and Addiction*. doi:Advance online publication DOI: 10.1007/s11469-011-9312-y.

McDonnell-Phillips Pty Ltd. (2005). *Analysis of gambler precommitment behaviour*. Melbourne: Victoria: Gambling Research Australia. Department of Justice.

McLaughlin, D., & Jinks, B. (2011). Online poker companies reach accord with U.S. on players' access to money. *Bloomberg News*. Retrieved from http://www.bloomberg.com/news/2011-04-20/online-poker-companies-reach-accord-with-u-s-on-players-access-to-money.html

McMillen, J. (2000). Online gambling: Challenges to national sovereignty and regulation. *Prometheus, 18*, 391–401.

McMillen, J. (2004) Internet gambling – a research perspective. DCITA Review of issues related to the commonwealth interactive gambling regulation

McMillen, J., &Woolley, R. (2003). Australian online gambling policy: A lost opportunity? *Pacific conference on I-gaming*, Alice Springs.

McMullan, J. L., & Rege, A. (2010). Online crime and internet gambling. *Journal of Gambling Issues, 24*, 54–85.

Meerkamper, E. (2006). *Decoding risk: Gambling attitudes and behaviours amongst youth in Nova Scotia*. Toronto: D-Code Inc.

Merten, M. (2011). Internet gambling rules soon. *i/O Scitech*. Retrieved from http://www.iol.co.za/scitech/technology/internet/internet-gambling-rules-soon-1.1118078

Microblogging, social networking still growing worldwide. (2011). *MarketingProfs*. Retrieved from http://www.marketingprofs.com/charts/2011/5891/microblogging-social-networking-still-growing-worldwide

Mihaylova, T., & Kairouz, S. (2010). *Risk factors in internet and non-internet gambling and video-game playing among university students*. 8th European Conference on Gambling and Policy Issues, Vienna, Austria.

Ministry of Community Development, Youth & Sports (2008). *Report of survey on participation in gambling activities among Singapore residents, 2008*. Singapore: Ministry of Community Development, Youth & Sports. Retrieved from http://app1.mcys.gov.sg/ResearchRoom/ResearchStatistics/SurveyonGamblingParticipationAmongSingaporeR.aspx

Miniwatts Marketing Group (2010). *World internet usage and population statistics.* Retrieved from http://www.internetworldstats.com/list4.htm#high

Miniwatts Marketing Group. (2011a). *Internet world stats.* Retrieved from http://www.internet worldstats.com/stats.htm

Miniwatts Marketing Group. (2011b). *New Facebook Stats for 2011 Q2.* Retrieved from http://www.internetworldstats.com/facebook.htm

Mobile gambling to capture more of market. (2011). *Online Casino Reports.* Retrieved from http://www.onlinecasinoreports.com/news/specialreports/2011/8/10/mobile-gambling-to-capture-more-of-market.php

Monaghan, S. (2008). *Internet and wireless gambling: A current profile.* Melbourne: Australian Gaming Council.

Monaghan, S. (2009a). Editorial – internet gambling: Not just a fad. *International Gambling Studies, 9,* 1–4.

Monaghan, S. (2009b). Responsible gambling strategies for internet gambling: The theoretical and empirical base of using pop-up messages to encourage self-awareness. *Computers in Human Behavior, 25,* 202–207.

Monaghan, S., & Blaszczynski, A. (2010a). Impact of mode of display and message content of responsible gambling signs for electronic gaming machines on regular gamblers. *Journal of Gambling Studies, 26,* 67–88.

Monaghan, S., & Blaszczynski, A. (2010b). Electronic gaming machine warning messages: Informative versus self-evaluation. *Journal of Psychology: Interdisciplinary & Applied, 144,* 83–96.

Monaghan, S., & Derevensky, J. (2008). An appraisal of the impact of the depiction of gambling in society on youth. *International Journal of Mental Health and Addiction, 6*(4), 537–550.

Monaghan, S., & Wood, R. T. A. (2010). Internet-based interventions for youth dealing with gambling problems. *International Journal of Adolescent Health and Medicine, 22*(1), 113–128.

Monaghan, S., Derevensky, J., & Sklar, A. (2009) Impact of gambling advertisements on children and adolescents: Policy recommendations to minimize harm. *Journal of Gambling Issues, 22,* 252–274. Retrieved from http://www.camh.net/egambling/issue22/06monaghan-derevensky.html

Moore, L. (2011). Class-action suit claims Full Tilt Poker kept users' money. *The Gazette.* Retrieved from http://www.montrealgazette.com/business/Class+action+suit+claims+Full+Tilt+Poker+kept+users+money/5381301/story.html

MORI/International Gaming Research Unit. (2006). *Under 16s and the National Lottery.* London: National Lottery Commission.

Motivation (2005). *Interactive and SMS or telephone gaming market monitor 2005.* Amsterdam, Netherlands. Retrieved from http://www.toezichtkansspelen.nl/information.html

National Centre for Academic Research into Gaming. (1999). *Project South Africa: Internet gaming and South Africa – Implications, costs & opportunities.* Cape Town: The National Gambling Board.

National Research Council. (1999). *Pathological gambling: A critical review.* Washington, DC: National Academy Press.

NCH. (2004). Children as young as eleven can set up gambling at the click of a button. Retrieved from http://www.nch.org.uk/information/index.php?i=77&r=288

Nelson, S., LaPlante, D., Peller, A., Schumann, A., LaBrie, R., & Shaffer, H. (2008). Real limits in the virtual world: Self-limiting behavior of internet gamblers. *Journal of Gambling Studies, 24,* 463–477.

Netherlands online plans criticized. (2011). *Global Gaming Business Magazine, 10*(10).

Nevada approves in-room gambling. (2011). *Global Gaming Business News, 9*(39).

New H2 eGaming dataset now available. (2011). *H2 Gambling Capital.* Retrieved from http://www.h2gc.com/news.php?article=New+H2+eGaming+Dataset+Now+Available

New Zealand looks at online lottery expansion. (2011). *Online-Casinos.com.* Retrieved from http://www.online-casinos.com/news/news1210744.asp

News Ltd reveals online gaming as next phase of micropayments strategy. (2009). *mUmBRELLA,* Retrieved from http://mumbrella.com.au/news-reveals-online-gaming-as-next-phase-of-micro-payments-strategy-12849

Nisbet, S. (2005). Responsible gambling features of card-based technologies. *International Journal of Mental Health and Addiction, 3*(2), 54–63.

O'Brien, R. (2011). Change in UK gambling law may hit company tax bills. *Reuters.* Retrieved from http://www.reuters.com/article/2011/07/14/britain-gambling-idUSL6E7IE20T20110714

Office of Public Sector Information. (2005). *Gambling Act.* London, UK: Author. Retrieved from http://www.opsi.gov.uk/ACTS/acts2005/20050019.htm

Olason, D. (2009). *Gambling and problem gambling studies among Nordic adults: Are they comparable?* 7th Nordic conference, Helsinki, Finland.

Olason, D. T., Kristjansdottir, E., Einarsdottir, H., Haraldsson, H., Bjarnason, G., & Derevensky, J. (2011). Internet gambling and problem gambling among 13 to 18 year old adolescents in Iceland. *International Journal of Mental Health and Addiction, 9*(3), 257–263.

Online Facebook betting game aiming at kids. (2011). *Herald Sun.* Retrieved from http://www.heraldsun.com.au/technology/online-facebook-betting-game-aiming-at-kids/story-fn7celvh-1226099361047

Online gambling strife on the rise. (2011). *Knox Leader.* Retrieved from http://knox-leader.whereilive.com.au/news/story/online-gambling-strife-on-the-rise/

Online gaming and entertainment company 2UP enters agreement to buy online pokies/slo. (2011). Retrieved from http://www.mycompanypr.com/online-gaming-and-entertainment-company-2up-enters-agreement-to-buy-online-pokiesslo/pr/10801/

Online sports betting in France drops 26.5%. (2011). *eGaming Review* Magazine. Retrieved from http://www.egrmagazine.com/news/1658042/online-sports-betting-in-france-drops-265.thtml

Opportunities in Indian E-gaming market. (2011). *Global betting & gaming consultants.* Retrieved from http://www.gbgc.com/2010/04/opportunity-in-indian-e-gaming-market/

Owens, M. D. (2010). There's an app for that (or soon will be): Smart phones, social networking and internet gambling. *Gaming Law Review, and Economics, 14*(3), 171–174.

PaddyPower buys into Australia online wagering market growing at 16% a year. (2010). *eCommerce Report.* Retrieved from http://www.ecommercereport.com.au/story126.php

Park, S., Je Cho, M., Jin Jeon, H., Woo Lee, H., Nam Bae, J., Ilk Park, J., et al. (2010). Prevalence, clinical correlations, comorbidities, and suicidal tendencies in pathological Korean gamblers: Results from the Korean epidemiologic catchment area study. *Social Psychiatry and Psychiatric Epidemiology, 45*(6), 621–629.

Parke, J., & Griffiths, M. (2001). Internet gambling: A small qualitative pilot study. Paper presented at the psychology and the internet conference, British Psychological Society, Farnborough, UK.

Parke, J., Rigbye, J., & Parke, A. (2008). *Cashless and card-based technologies in gambling: A review of the literature.* Report for the Gambling Commission, Salford: University of Salford

Parness, N. (2010). OLG to bring online gaming to Ontario in 2012. *CTV News,* Retrieved from http://www.ctv.ca/CTVNews/Canada/20100810/ontario-online-gambling-duncan-100810/

Pasadeos, Y. (1990). Perceived informativeness of and irritation with local advertising. *Journalism Quarterly, 67,* 35–39.

Paul Budd Communication. (2010). *Digital media – social networks & gaming insights.* Bucketty: Paul Budde Communication.

Pavalko, R. M. (2004). Gambling and public policy. *Public Integrity, 6,* 333–3348.

Peppin, J. (2011a). Online gambling problems in Scandinavia. *Casino Advisor.* Retrieved from http://www.casinoadvisor.com/online-gambling-problems-in-scandinavia-news-item.html

Peppin, J. (2011b). Online gambling crackdown in Asia. *Casino Advisor.* Retrieved from http://www.casinoadvisor.com/online-gambling-crackdown-in-asia-news-item.html

Petrolli, J. (2011). Betting shop: Controversy triggered by New Zealand's National Lottery Commission. *Boomakers Inc.* Retrieved from http://www.bookmakersinc.co.uk/betting-site/betting-shop-controversy-triggeredbynewzealandsnationallotterycommission/

Petry, N. (2005). *Pathological gambling: Etiology, comorbidity and treatment.* Washington, DC: American Psychological Association.

Petry, N. (2006). Internet gambling: An emerging concern in family practice medicine? *Family Practice, 23*(4), 421–426.

Petry, N., & Weinstock, J. (2007). Internet gambling is common in college students and associated with poor mental health. *The American Journal on Addictions, 16*, 325–330.

Pew Internet & American life Project. (2001). *Teenage life online: The rise of the instant-message generation and the Internet's impact on friendships and family relationship.* Retrieved from http://ww.pewinternet.org/

Pew Internet & American life Project. (2009). *Generations Online in 2009.* Retrieved from http://ww.pewinternet.org/

Pew Research Center. (2006). Gambling: As the take rises so does public concern. Retrieved from http://pewresearch.org

Phillips, J. G., & Blaszczynski, A. (2010). *Gambling and the impact of new and emerging technologies and associated products.* Port Melbourne: Gambling Research Australia. Retrieved from http://www.gamblingresearch.org.au/CA256DB1001771FB/page/GRA+Research+Reports-Gambling+and+the+impact+of+new+and+emerging+technologies+and+associated+products?OpenDocument&1=35-GRA+Research+Reports~&2=0-

Pilieci, V. (2011). Gambling on gaming at home: Virgin, EA deal takes home consoles to a new level with online wagering. *Ottawa Citizen.* Retrieved from www.responsiblegambling.org/articles/Gambling_on_gaming_at_home.pdf

Ploeckl, B. (2011). The EU responds to Germany's draft legislation. *World Online Gambling Law Report, 10*(7), 1.

Post, K. (2010). Online-gambling ban enforced as House works to lift it. *Press of Atlantic City.* Retrieved from http://www.pressofatlanticcity.com/business/article_7f9cf839-99e8-5016-b9e2-7194d99d5ab9.html

Powell, J., Hardoon, K., Derevensky, J., & Gupta, R. (1996). *Gambling and risk taking behaviour amongst university students.* 10th National Conference on Gambling Behavior, Chicago.

PricewaterhouseCoopers (2010). *Playing to win.* Retrieved from http://www.pwc.com/e&m

PricewaterhouseCoopers. (2011). *Global gaming outlook.* Retrieved from http://www.pwc.com/en_GX/gx/entertainment-media/publications/global-gaming-outlook.jhtml

Problem Gambling Foundation. (2011). More youth seeking help for problem gambling. *Scoop Independent News.* Retrieved from http://www.scoop.co.nz/stories/GE1102/S00001/more-youth-seeking-help-for-problem-gambling.htm

Productivity Commission. (2010). *Gambling*, Report no: 50, Canberra.

Pulsipher, I. (2005). Counting on gambling. *State Legislatures*, 24–26.

Rainone, G., & Gallati, R. (2007). *Gambling behaviors and problem gambling among adolescents in New York State: Initial findings from the 2006 OASAS School Survey.* New York: New York Office of Alcoholism and Substance Abuse Services.

Ranade, S., Bailey, S., & Harvey, A. (2006). *A literature review and survey of statistical sources on remote gambling.* London: RSeconsulting.

Reichel, B. (2010). *The future of interactive wagering.* Sydney: Gambling Reform Summit.

Reichheld, F. F., & Schefter, P. (2000). E-loyalty: Your secret weapon on the web. *Harvard Business Review, 78*, 105–113.

Reith, G. (2006). *Research on the social impacts of gambling: Final report.* Edinburgh: Scottish Executive Social Research.

Remmers, P. (2006). *The social outlook of remote and e-gambling: Are we serious?* 13th international conference on gambling & risk taking. Nevada: Lake Tahoe.

Report, World Online Gambling Law. (2011). EU takes stance against several national gaming draft provisions. *World Online Gambling Law Report, 10*(7), 1.

Reuters. (2001). *Hackers heaven: Online gambling.* Retrieved from http://www.cbsnews.com/stories/2001/09/10/tech/main310567.html

Reuters. (2008). "Irresponsible" online gambling advert banned. *Reuters U.K. Edition.* Retrieved from http://uk.reuters.com/article/2008/04/23/uk-britain-gambling-idUKELK33050220080423

Reuters. (2011). Dutch government seeks to allow online gambling. *Reuters U.S. Edition.* Retrieved from http://www.reuters.com/article/2011/03/19/us-netherlands-gambling-idUSTRE72I20F20110319

Rodda, S., & Cowie, M. (2005). *Evaluation of electronic gaming machine harm minimisation in Victoria: Final report*. Melbourne, Australia: Office of Gaming and Racing, Victorian Government Department of Justice

Rogge, K., & Ukkelberg, A. (2010). *Playing habits and problems in population 2010*. Oslo: Synovate.

Rose, I. N. (2008). Regulators punt on proposed internet gambling regulations. *Gaming Law Review, 12*, 1–4.

Rose, I. N. (2010). Mergers and acquisitions: Why so many, why now? *IGaming Business, 61(March/April)*, 54–55.

Rose, I. N. (2011). Land-based to online. *Gambling and the Law*. Retrieved from http://www.gamblingandthelaw.com/columns/314-land-based-to-online.html

Rovell, D. (2011). Insider breakdown of poker's black Friday/ *CNBC*. Retrieved from http://www.cnbc.com/id/42649117

Roy Morgan Research. (2010). *Gambling monitor*. Sydney: Roy Morgan Research.

Roy Morgan Research. (2011). *Gambling monitor*. Sydney: Roy Morgan Research.

RSeConsulting. (2006) *A literature review and survey of statistical sources on remote gambling: Final report*. Retrieved from http://www.culture.gov.uk/NR/rdonlyres/89D59ABD-A1F6-4106-B922-2293997EF841/0/RemoteGamblingAppendix_RSeReport.pdf

Ryan, J. (2011). FBI cracks down on internet gambling companies. *ABC News*. Retrieved from http://abcnews.go.com/Technology/internet-gambling-companies-indicted-fraud-money-laundering/story?id=13389751

Sandman, J. (2008). Momentum builds against Internet gambling prohibition. *Casino & Gaming International, 2*, 23–26.

Sandven, U. (2007). *The preset situation in Norway*. 6th Nordic conference on gambling and policy issue, Copenhagen.

Schellinck, T., & Schrans, T. (2007). *VLT player tracking system*. Nova Scotia: Focal Research.

Screen Digest. (2009). *Bingo in the digital age: Global market assessment and forecasts*. Retrieved from http://www.screendigest.com/reports/09bingointhedigitalage/pdf/SD-09-03-3DBingoInTheDigitalAge/view.html

Second U.S casino to go online with Aristocrat. (2011). *Gaming Intelligence*. Retrieved from http://www.gamingintelligence.com/business/13473-second-us-casino-to-go-online-with-aristocrat

Shaffer, H., & Korn, D. (2002). Gambling and related mental disorders: A public health analysis. *Annual Review of Public Health, 23*, 171–212.

Shaffer, H. J., & Martin, R. (2011). Disordered gambling: Etiology, trajectory, and clinical considerations. *Annual Review of Clinical Psychology, 7*, 485–510.

Shapira, N., Goldsmith, T., Keck, P., Khosla, U., & McElroy, S. (2001). Psychiatric features of individuals with problematic internet use. *Journal of Affective Disorders, 57*, 267–272.

Shelat, B., & Egger, F. N. (2002). *What makes people trust online gambling sites?* CHI 2002: Changing the World, Changing Ourselves. Minneapolis, Minnesota, Retrieved from http://portal.acm.org/citation.cfm?id=506631

Smeaton, M., & Griffiths, M. (2004). Internet gambling and social responsibility: An exploratory study. *CyberPsychology and Behaviour, 7*(1), 49–57.

Smith, P. (2011). Lack of resources costs $1m in fines. *The Australian*, Retrieved from http://www.theaustralian.com.au/news/sport/lack-of-resources-costs-1m-in-fines/story-e6frg7mf-1226095581505

Smith, G. J., Schopflocher, D. P., el-Guebaly, N., Casey, D., Hodgins, D. C., Willams, R. J., et al. (2011). Community attitudes towards legalised gambling in Alberta. *International Gambling Studies, 11*, 57–79.

South Australian Centre for Economic Studies. (2008). *Social and economic impact study into gambling in Tasmania 2008: Fact Sheets*. Retrieved from http://www.dhhs.tas.gov.au/__data/assets/pdf_file/0015/33027/Vol_2_Fact_Sheets.pdf

Sportsman adds Australian Open to live stream service. (2011). *Gaming Intelligence*. Retrieved from http://gamingintelligence.com/marketing/13410-sportsman-media-adds-australian-open-to-live-stream-service

State aid: Commission clears Danish online gambling dues. (2011). *European Commission Press release IP/11/1048.* Retrieved from http://europa.eu/rapid/showInformation.do

Statistics Canada. (2010). *CANSIM individual and household internet use.* Retrieved from http://www40.statcan.gc.ca/l01/cst01/comm32a-eng.htm

Stewart, D., Ropes & Gray, L.L.P. (2006). *An analysis of internet gambling and its policy implications.* American Gaming Association. Retrieved from www.americangaming.org/assets/files/studies/wpaper_internet_0531.pdf

Story, M., & French, S. (2004). Food advertising and marketing directed at children and adolescents in the US. *International Journal of Behavioral Nutrition and Physical Activity, 1.* Retrieved from http://www.ijbnpa.org/content/pdf/1479-5868-1-3.pdf

Stradbrooke, S. (2011). China's new internet watchdog: Chinese bet online twice as much as Yanks. *Calvin Ayre.com.* Retrieved from http://calvinayre.com/2011/05/06/business/china-new-internet-gambling-watchdog/

Stymne, A. (2008). *Motives behind and effects of state-owned Netpoker.* Östersund: Swedish National Institute of Public Health.

Suggett, R. (2011). Apps versus websites. *EGaming Review Magazine.* Retrieved from http://www.egrmagazine.com/blog/1678172/apps-versus-websites.thtml

Survey: Growth in online gaming boosting IoM economy. (2011). *Gaming intelligence.* Retrieved from http://www.gamingintelligence.com/business/11941-survey-growth-in-online-gaming-boosting-iom-economy

Svensson, J., & Romild, R. (2011). Incident Internet gambling in Sweden: Results from the Swedish longitudinal gambling study. *International Gambling Studies, 11,* 257–375.

Swartz, J. (2005). Online gambling has hit the jackpot. USA Today.

Swedish National Institute of Public Health (2011). *Swedish Longitudinal Gambling Study, Report No. 3.* Östersund, Sweden: Swedish National Institute of Public Health. Retrieved from http://www.fhi.se/en/About-FHI/Contact-information/

Talisma. (2007). *Customer service audit of the online gambling industry.* Retrieved from http://www.talisma.com/tal_lp/default.aspx?id=1220&ac=WPDL.EU.Rpt.og.0108.web

Taylor, L. (2010). Why social media gaming is big business for your business. *Social Media Examiner.* Retrieved from http://www.socialmediaexaminer.com/why-social-media-gaming-is-big-business-for-your-business/

The Daily Telegraph set to offer online casino games. (2011). *Gaming Intelligence.* Retrieved from http://gamingintelligence.com/marketing/12907-the-daily-telegraph-set-to-offer-online-casino-games

The Impact of the FullTilt.com Site Closure – The First Look. (2011). *H2 gambling capital.* Retrieved from http://www.h2gc.com/news.php?article=The+Impact+of+the+FullTilt.com+Site+Closure+%96+The+First+Look

Toce-Gerstein, M., & Gerstein, D. (2007). Questionnaire design: The art of a stylized conversation. In G. Smith, D. Hodgins, & R. Williams (Eds.), *Research and measurement issues in gambling studies* (pp. 55–86). Burlington: Academic.

Tolchard, B., Thomas, L., & Battersby, M. (2006). Single-session exposure therapy for problem gambling: A single-case experimental design. *Behavioral Change, 23,* 148–55.

Toneatto, T., & Ladouceur, R. (2003). Treatment of pathological gambling: A critical review of the literature. *Psychology of Addictive Behaviors, 17*(4), 284–292.

Totalizator Regulation. (2005). Retrieved from http://www.legislation.nsw.gov.au

Tromp, S. (2011). In BC, we're losing our gambling fever. *TheTyee.ca.* Retrieved from http://thetyee.ca/News/2011/02/17/LosingGamblingFever/

Turner, E. N. (2008). Games, gambling and gambling problems. In M. Zangeneh, A. Blaszczynski, & N. E. Turner (Eds.), *The pursuit of winning: Problem gambling theory, research and treatment* (pp. 33–64). Berlin/Heidelberg/New York: Springer.

Twoway Interactive Entertainment. (2011). *Cash flow statement and investor update.* ASX: TTV.

UK Press Association. (2011). Betfair profits from gadget trends. *Press Association.* Retrieved from http://www.google.com/hostednews/ukpress/article/ALeqM5iOzt5xWDa6Yk2dJnIRm-sj64XVXA?docId=N0222101315307497049A

United States Attorney's Office. (2008) *Twelve charged in multimillion dollar internet gambling operation*. Accessed from http://newyork.fbi.gov/dojpressrel/pressrel08/internetgambling 010708.htm

United States General Accounting Office. (2002). Internet gambling: An overview of the issues. Government Reports.

University of Sydney. (2011). Internet adds to gambling woes. *Science Alert*. Retrieved from http:// www.sciencealert.com.au/news/20111503-21947.html

Urban, G. L., Sultan, F., & Qualls, W. (1999). *Design and evaluation of a trust based advisor on the Internet*. Working paper, Massachusetts Institute of Technology. Retrieved from http:// ebusiness.mit.edu/research/papers/Urban.pdf

Vardi, N. (2011). How the Las Vegas casino companies became the champions of online poker in America. *Forbes*. Retrieved from http://www.forbes.com/sites/nathanvardi/2011/09/30/how-the-las-vegas-casino-companies-became-the-champions-of-online-poker-in-america/

Victorian Commission for Gambling Regulation. (2011). Media release. Retrieved from http:// www.vcgr.vic.gov.au

Vlaemminck, P., & De Wael, P. (2003). The European Union regulatory approach of online gambling and its impact on the global gaming industry. *Gaming Law Review, 7*, 177–184.

Volberg, R. A. (2010). *Epidemiological study of the prevalence of pathological gambling in the adult population of Catalonia 2007-2008* 8th European conference on gambling studies and policy issues, Vienna Austria. Retrieved from http://www.easg.org/website/conference.cfm?id =13&cid=13&section=AGENDA&day=2

Volberg, R. A., Nysse-Carris, K. L., & Gerstein, D. R. (2006). 2006 California problem gambling prevalence survey. Final report. Submitted to the California Department of Alcohol and drug Problems, Office of Problem and Pathological Gambling.

Wardle, H., Moody, A., Griffiths, M., Orford, J., & Volberg, R. (2011a). Defining the online gambler and patterns of behaviour integration: Evidence from the British Gambling Prevalence Survey 2010. *International Gambling Studies, 11*, 339–356.

Wardle, H., Moody, A., Spence, S., Orford, J., Volberg, R., Jotangia, D., & Dobbie, F. (2011b). *British gambling prevalence survey 2010*. London: National Centre for Social Research.

Welte, J., Barnes, G., Tidwell, M., & Hoffman, J. (2009). The association of form of gambling with problem gambling among American youth. *Psychology of Addictive Behaviors, 23*, 105–12.

White, A. (2011), Germany's draft gambling rules need to be changed, EU says. *Bloomberg*. Retrieved from http://www.bloomberg.com/news/2011-07-18/germany-s-draft-gambling-rules-need-to-be-changed-eu-says.html

Willems, M. (2011). UK outlines license scheme for foreign-based operators. *World Online Gambling Law Report, 10*(7), 1.

Williams, R., & Wood, R. (2007). *Internet gambling: A comprehensive review and synthesis of the literature*. Report prepared for the Ontario Problem Gambling Research Centre, Guelph.

Williams, S. (2011). US Government clampdown on gambling targets online bingo operators. *Bingo News*. Retrieved from http://bestbingospots.com/bingo-news/1767/us-government-clampdown-on-gambling-targets-online-bingo-operators/

Wilsenach, A. (2011). *The ever changing faces of Internet gambling regulation*. Discovery 2011, Ottawa. Retrieved from http://www.responsiblegambling.org/en/programs/events-discovery-2011. cfm#1

Winder, D. (2011). Phishing for chips: Why the online gambling industry is odds-on to beat cybercrime. *InfoSecurity, March/April*, 32–34

Wingfield, N., Anupreeta, D., & Chon, G. (2011). Zynga preparing to file IPO. *The Wall Street Journal*. Retrieved from http://online.wsj.com/article/SB10001424052702304447804576414111297459234.html

Wohl, M. & Pellizzari, P. (2011). *Player tools, do they work? New research and implications for operators*. Nova Scotia Gaming Corporation Responsible Gambling Conference, Halifax, NS. Retrieved from http://www.responsiblegamblingns.ca/presentations/

Wood, R. T. A. (2010). *Review of the Espacejeux responsible gambling strategy*. Loto Quebec. Retrieved from http://lotoquebec.com/corporatif/nav/en/news-room/documentation-centre

Wood, R. T. A., & Griffiths, M. D. (2008). Why Swedish people play online poker and factors that can increase or decrease trust in poker web sites: A qualitative investigation. *Journal of Gambling Issues, 21*, 80–97.

Wood, R. T. A., Griffiths, M. D., & Parke, J. (2007). The acquisition, development, and maintenance of online poker playing in a student sample. *Cyberpsychology & Behavior, 10*, 354–361.

Wood, R., & Williams, R. (2007). Problem gambling on the internet: Implications for internet gambling policy in North America. *New Media & Society, 9*, 520–542.

Wood, R., Williams, R., & Lawton, P. (2007). Why do Internet gamblers prefer online versus land-based venues: Some preliminary findings and implications. *Journal of Gambling Issues, 20*, 235–252.

Wood, R., & Williams, R. (2010). *Internet gambling: Prevalence, patterns, problems, and policy options*, Final report prepared for the Ontario Problem Gambling Research Centre, Guelph.

Wood, R., & Williams, R. (2011). A comparative profile of the internet gambler: Demographic characteristics, game play patterns, and problem gambling status. *New Media & Society, 13*, 1123–1141; Wood, R., Williams, R., & Lawton, P. (2007). Why do internet gamblers prefer online versus land-based venues: Some preliminary findings and implications. *Journal of Gambling Issues, 20*.

Woodruff, C., & Gregory, S. (2005). Profile of internet gamblers: Betting on the future. *UNLV Gaming Research & Review Journal, 9*, 1–14.

Woolley, R. (2003). Mapping internet gambling: Emerging modes of online participation in wagering and sports betting. *International Gambling Studies, 3*, 3–21.

Worldwide Smartphone Market Expected to Grow 55% in 2011 and Approach Shipments of One Billion in 2015. (2011). *International Data Corporation*, Press Release. Retrieved from http://www.idc.com/getdoc.jsp?containerId=prUS22871611

Xuan, Z., & Shaffer, H. J. (2009). How do gamblers end gambling: Longitudinal analysis of Internet gambling behaviors prior to account closure due to gambling related problems. *Journal of Gambling Studies, 25*, 239–252.

Young, K. (1998a). *Caught in the net*. New York: Wiley.

Young, K. (1998b). Internet addiction: The emergence of a new clinical disorder. *Cyberpsychology & Behavior, 1*, 237–244.

Lightning Source UK Ltd.
Milton Keynes UK
UKOW04f0926080813

215017UK00003B/140/P